Karolyn

Patient Outcomes in Pediatric Nursing

Grace R. Whitis, RN, PhD
Professor of Nursing
Arkansas State University
State University, Arkansas

Patricia Iyer, RN, MSN, CNA
President
Patricia Iyer Associates
Stockton, New Jersey

Springhouse Corporation
Springhouse, Pennsylvania

Staff

EXECUTIVE DIRECTOR, EDITORIAL
Stanley Loeb

SENIOR PUBLISHER, TRADE AND TEXTBOOKS
Minnie B. Rose, RN, BSN, MEd

ART DIRECTOR
John Hubbard

CLINICAL EDITOR
Patricia Kardish Fischer, RN, BSN

EDITORS
Nancy Priff (senior editor), Rafaela Ellis, Cathy Somer

ASSOCIATE ACQUISITIONS EDITOR
Caroline Lemoine

COPY EDITORS
Debra Davis, Tracy Ginnona, Barbara Hodgson

DESIGNERS
Stephanie Peters (associate art director), Cindy Marczuk

EDITORIAL ASSISTANT
Louise Quinn

MANUFACTURING
Deborah Meiris (director), Anna Brindisi, Kate Davis, T.A. Landis

The clinical procedures described and recommended in this publication are based on currently accepted clinical theory and practice and on consultation with medical and nursing authorities. Nevertheless, they cannot be considered absolute and universal recommendations. For individual application, recommendations must be considered in light of the client's clinical condition and, before administration of new or infrequently used drugs, in light of the latest package-insert information. The authors and the publisher disclaim responsibility for any adverse effects resulting directly or indirectly from the suggested procedures, from any undetected errors, or from the reader's misunderstanding of the text.

Printed in the United States of America. For information, write Springhouse Corporation, 1111 Bethlehem Pike, P.O. Box 908, Springhouse, PA 19477-0908.

PTOUTPEDS-011094

A member of the Reed Elsevier plc group

Library of Congress Cataloging-in-Publication Data

Whitis, Grace R.
Patient outcomes in pediatric nursing/Grace R. Whitis. Patricia Iyer.
p. cm.
Includes bibliographical references and index.
1. Pediatric nursing.
2. Outcome assessment (Medical care)
I. Iyer, Patricia W. II. Title.
[DNLM: 1. Pediatric Nursing--methods.
2. Outcome and Process Assessment (HealthCare)
WY 159 W613p 1994]
RJ245.W476 1994
610.73'62--dc20
DNLM/DLC

ISBN 0-87434-702-5 94-26705 CIP

Contents

RESPIRATORY DISORDERS

APPENDICES, SELECTED REFERENCES, AND INDEX

Acknowledgments and Dedication

This book is the result of the efforts of a number of persons. Style and content editors have worked patiently with the series author, Patricia Iyer, RN, MSN, CNA, to polish the final product. The author wishes to thank the series author for gently guiding the product to completion.

The author also gratefully acknowledges the thorough expert reviews provided by the following:

Linda Hood Pehl, RN,C, PhD
Professor of Nursing
University of Mary Hardin-Baylor
Belton, Texas

Kathie J. Dalton, RN,P, MSN
Assistant Professor of Nursing
Arkansas State University
Jonesboro, Arkansas

JoAnne Kardish Resnic, RN, BSN
Clinical Administrator
Paidos Health Care Incorporated
Paoli, Pennsylvania

Dedication

To my family
Robert E. Whitis, husband
Jay K. Whitis, son
Jennifer A. Whitis, daughter
for loving support and for being there
and to the memory of my parents
Allan and Jewel Richardson

Preface

Patient Outcomes in Pediatric Nursing helps the nurse fulfill the roles of teacher, advanced practitioner, and quality assurance manager by focusing on outcomes that can be used to measure and direct care. Organized primarily by body system, each section of the text includes entries on common conditions, which are alphabetized for easy access. Each entry follows a standard format:

• *Definition* that describes the condition or health care concern.

• *Nursing diagnosis* that focuses the plan of care.

• *Desired patient outcome* that reflects the nursing diagnosis and directs the outcome measurement criteria.

• *Outcome measurement criteria* set the nursing standard for ensuring quality assurance.

• *Key interventions* reflect essential nursing activities to help children stay healthy or move toward health; interventions may be independent, collaborative, or dependent.

Patient Outcomes in Pediatric Nursing includes appendices on the NANDA taxonomy of nursing diagnoses and common nursing diagnoses in pediatric care. Its selected references provide resources for additional information.

This book is invaluable for developing plans of care, documenting patient care, ensuring quality care, and developing standard outcomes.

Burns

Damage to and loss of dermal or underlying tissues, or both, as a result of thermal, chemical, electrical, or solar ray contact.

NURSING DIAGNOSIS

Ineffective airway clearance related to upper airway inflammation and edema

DESIRED PATIENT OUTCOME

The child will maintain a patent airway

Outcome measurement criteria

- ☐ Patent airway
- ☐ Age-appropriate vital signs
- ☐ Absence of obvious signs of respiratory difficulty, such as stridor, retractions, and flaring
- ☐ Age-appropriate blood gas levels
- ☐ Absence of injury caused by seizures
- ☐ Alertness

Key interventions

- Determine airway patency and the presence of a pulse; administer cardiopulmonary resuscitation (CPR) if needed.
- Assess the child carefully for signs of burns or inhalation injury, such as burns on face or neck; dyspnea; edema of mouth and nose tissues; history of exposure to open flames or to smoke- or vapor-filled spaces; hoarseness or

coughing; singed hair, eyelashes, or eyebrows; and soot on face or in nose or mouth.

- Take seizure precautions if the child has inhaled poisonous or irritating fumes or is hypoxic.
- Intubate the child and monitor vital signs carefully for 24 hours if inhalation injury is suspected; suction endotracheal tube as needed.
- Administer humidified oxygen via a tent and place the child in semi-Fowler's position, if not intubated.
- Determine blood oxygen, carbon dioxide, and carbon monoxide levels.
- Assess the extent of the burn using age-related body surface area charts.
- Assess burn depth by using appropriate burn classifications: superficial (first-degree), partial-thickness (second-degree), and full-thickness (third-degree). Assess burn severity by determining the percentage of each burn classification and considering the type of burn, age of child, and other complicating factors.

NURSING DIAGNOSIS

Fluid volume deficit related to burn-induced fluid loss and interstitial fluid shift

DESIRED PATIENT OUTCOME

The child will display sufficient fluid volume

Outcome measurement criteria

- ☐ Moist mucous membranes
- ☐ Adequate urine output (1 to 2 ml/kg/hour)
- ☐ Age-appropriate vital signs
- ☐ Age-appropriate urine specific gravity
- ☐ Capillary refill time of less than 2 seconds

Key interventions

- Strictly monitor the child's fluid intake and output. Measure oral and I.V. intake as appropriate and output, including urine from catheter, nasogastric secretions, and vomitus. Also weigh saturated linens.
- Note urine color; obtain an order to increase the fluid rate if urine is red or tea-colored.
- Measure urine specific gravity, check vital signs, and check capillary refill time every hour during the first 72 hours.
- Note the child's level of consciousness (LOC) and check mucous membranes for moistness every hour.
- Weigh the child and check serum pH every 4 hours.
- Assess for edema and describe its location.
- Provide mouth care every 4 hours and as necessary.
- Monitor the I.V. site and drip rate.

NURSING DIAGNOSIS

Altered nutrition: less than body requirements, related to poor intake and increased metabolic needs

DESIRED PATIENT OUTCOME

The child will have adequate nutritional intake to meet body requirements

Outcome measurement criteria

- ☐ Age-appropriate weight
- ☐ Laboratory serum values that indicate adequate protein and glucose intake
- ☐ Adequate nutrient intake for the child's age
- ☐ Verbalization by the child's parents of the importance of adequate nutritional intake

Key interventions

- Weigh the child daily at the same time, using the same scale, and with the child wearing the same amount of clothing each time.
- Separate the time of meals from the time of dressing changes and other potentially unpleasant procedures, when possible.
- Administer prescribed vitamins and minerals.
- Check for bowel sounds before feeding the child.
- Develop a contract with the child (if age-appropriate) and reward the child for increased oral intake.
- Offer favorite foods and drinks in frequent, small meals. Offer high-protein and high-carbohydrate snacks, encourage the family to bring the child's favorite foods from home, and permit the child to choose between equally acceptable foods.
- Consult and collaborate with a dietitian to implement a plan to meet the child's nutritional needs. Explain to the parents and child (if age-appropriate) the importance of food intake to healing.
- Blend food and feed the child through a nasogastric tube if food intake is minimal and the child's weight is decreasing.

NURSING DIAGNOSIS

Impaired physical mobility related to acute pain secondary to the injury and therapy

DESIRED PATIENT OUTCOME

The child will maintain normal range of motion (ROM) and joint function

Outcome measurement criteria

☐ Full ROM in affected joints

- ☐ Performance of age-appropriate self-care activities
- ☐ Report of minimal discomfort during activities that require joint ROM and function
- ☐ Documentation on children's pain scale of progressive decrease in discomfort

Key interventions

- Involve the child in age-appropriate self-care activities, such as eating, bathing, and dressing.
- Encourage the child to play games that require movement of affected joints.
- Assess for pain using the age-appropriate children's pain scale.
- Provide scheduled pain medication for ongoing discomfort.
- Provide I.V. pain medication 15 minutes before strenuous joint exercises.
- Provide age-appropriate diversionary activities during less strenuous joint exercises. Have the family bring familiar games and toys from home.
- Splint and position joints for comfort during rest and sleep.

NURSING DIAGNOSIS

High risk for infection related to loss of skin secondary to a burn

DESIRED PATIENT OUTCOME

The child will remain free from infection

Outcome measurement criteria

- ☐ Axillary temperature at or below 98° F (36.7° C); oral or tympanic temperature at or below 99° F (37.2° C)

- ☐ Absence of signs of infection in wounds
- ☐ Absence of signs of infection in lung fields
- ☐ Removal of sources of possible infection
- ☐ Absence of flora changes in wound cultures
- ☐ White blood cell (WBC) count within normal range for the child's age

Key interventions

- Administer tetanus prophylaxis as prescribed.
- Use universal precautions when contact with blood or body fluids is possible.
- Clean wounds and nearby skin thoroughly while the child is under anesthesia or sedated by I.V. analgesia.
- Assess wounds at each dressing change.
- Apply topical antibacterial creams and dressings as prescribed.
- Thoroughly clean the perineal area daily; change the indwelling urinary (Foley) catheter weekly.
- Maintain appropriate hydration.
- Assess lung fields every 2 hours after the first 72 hours.
- Assess vital signs every 2 hours after the first 72 hours.
- Assess the child's LOC every 2 hours after the first 72 hours.
- Use sterile gloves, linens, and equipment if in contact with burned areas.
- Obtain cultures from various wound sites every other day.
- Obtain blood, urine, and sputum cultures if the child's temperature is above 101° F (38.3° C).
- Monitor the child's WBC count.
- Check for bowel sounds.

- Advise all people coming into contact with the child to wash their hands thoroughly.
- Screen visitors to eliminate those with respiratory or other infections.

NURSING DIAGNOSIS

Altered family processes related to the child's hospitalization and probable long-term rehabilitation

DESIRED PATIENT OUTCOME

The family will cope effectively with the child's hospitalization and rehabilitation

Outcome measurement criteria

- ☐ Verbalization by the family of feelings of guilt or anger regarding the child's burns
- ☐ Verbalization by the family of feelings about the child's long-term care
- ☐ Verbalization by the family of effects of the situation on other family members' plans for the future
- ☐ Use by the parents of available community resources to ease financial and other stresses associated with the child's care
- ☐ Participation of family members in the child's care
- ☐ Involvement of parents in a support group

Key interventions

- Arrange for the parents to meet with a social worker to discuss community resources that may be available to assist the family.
- Reassure the family that everything possible is being done for the child.

- Encourage family members to talk about the burn incident, their feelings of guilt or anger, and their concerns about the burn's effects on the family's future.
- Provide information on current hospitalization and probable rehabilitation care.
- Encourage family members to ask questions about hospital procedures and care provided for the child.
- Encourage at least one family member to visit the child as often as possible and to participate in care.
- Establish a routine to give the child a sense of structure and consistency.

NURSING DIAGNOSIS

High risk for injury related to lack of knowledge about preventing burns

DESIRED PATIENT OUTCOME

The child will experience no additional, preventable, serious burns during childhood

Outcome measurement criteria

- ☐ Verbalization by the parents and the child (if age-appropriate) of safety measures to prevent burns
- ☐ Verbalization by the parents of immediate first-aid measures for burns
- ☐ Verbalization by the child (if age-appropriate) of actions to take in case of fire or burns

Key interventions

- Teach the parents and child how to prevent burns. Suggest turning pot handles away from stove edges; setting the hot water heater on 120° F (48.8° C) or lower; refusing to allow children to turn on sink or bathtub faucets; dressing infants and young children in flame-retardant sleepwear; using plug covers on electrical outlets; placing electrical cords out of children's sight and reach; providing barriers to hot stoves, open-flame heaters, and similar equipment; avoiding flammables for cleaning; and locking flammables, matches, chemicals, and caustics in cabinets.

- Assess the home environment for fire safety, ensuring that sockets are not overloaded with extension cords, electrical cords are not frayed or damaged, flammables are not stored near open flames, functioning smoke detectors are located near the kitchen and bedrooms, and smoke detector batteries are checked routinely.
- Teach the child actions to take in case of fire or burns, such as learning an escape route from the home and using it in case of fire, calling the emergency response number or 911 from a neighbor's house or nearby phone, crawling on the floor if the room becomes smoke-filled, and rolling on the ground or floor to put out a fire if clothes are burning.
- Teach first-aid measures to use in case of burns. Advise the child and family members to stop the burning process by submerging burns in cool water and removing hot clothing. In case of electrical burns, advise family members to turn off the electricity or use a wooden object to separate the victim from the current, perform CPR if needed, and call emergency medical personnel. Advise the child and family members to flush chemical burns with water; to cover serious burns with a lint-free, clean cloth (do not apply ointment); and to take the child to the emergency department.

Childhood communicable diseases

Illnesses common during infancy and childhood that are transmitted directly or indirectly from one person to another.

NURSING DIAGNOSIS

High risk for fluid volume deficit related to fever or decreased oral intake

DESIRED PATIENT OUTCOME

The child will maintain adequate hydration

Outcome measurement criteria

- ☐ Axillary temperature at or below 98° F (36.7° C); oral or tympanic temperature at or below 99° F (37.2° C)
- ☐ Elastic skin turgor
- ☐ Age-appropriate fluid intake and output
- ☐ Flat (not depressed) fontanel, if patent
- ☐ Stable weight at pre-illness level
- ☐ Age-appropriate urine specific gravity

Key interventions

- Tell the parents to take the child's temperature every 4 hours or more often if needed.
- Explain to the parents that they may safely use an axillary or a tympanic thermometer for children of all ages or an oral thermometer if the child is school-age or older and can cooperate.
- Advise the parents to wash their hands before taking the child's temperature.

- Teach the parents to properly prepare the thermometer by shaking a mercury thermometer's reading below 96° F (35.6° C) and by inserting the probe tip of an electronic or a tympanic thermometer into a disposable cover.
- Teach the parents to insert the thermometer properly. Advise them to place an axillary thermometer in the child's axilla and then hold the arm against the child's body; to place the bulb of an oral thermometer under and to the side of the child's tongue, cautioning the child to close the lips but not to bite down on the thermometer; and to place the covered probe tip of the tympanic thermometer into the opening of the child's external auditory canal.
- Tell the parents to hold an axillary thermometer in place for 4 minutes (for a mercury thermometer) or until a beep is heard (for an electronic thermometer); to hold an oral thermometer in place for 3 minutes (mercury thermometer) or until a beep is heard (electronic thermometer); and to activate the scan on a tympanic thermometer and watch for the temperature to appear on the display.
- Teach the parents how to read the thermometer. Advise those using a mercury thermometer to hold the nonbulb end and slowly rotate it until a wide silver band appears, revealing the temperature reading at the right end. Explain to those using electronic thermometers to watch for the digital readout. Advise those using tympanic thermometers to watch the readout display and check the manufacturer's instructions about the need to retake the temperature.
- Caution the parents to clean the thermometer after each use. Advise them to wash the mercury thermometer with soap and cool water and store it out of children's reach and to discard the disposable cover of an electronic or a tympanic thermometer and replace the thermometer in the base unit.

- Administer medication, such as acetaminophen, as prescribed by the primary care practitioner (usually for temperature at or above 101° F [38.3° C]); avoid using aspirin unless directed by the primary care practitioner because of the risk of Reye's syndrome.
- Give the child favorite fluids or clear liquid foods, such as flavored gelatin, shaved ice, or a frozen pop, every hour (or more often if the child is willing).
- Place minimal clothing on the child, being careful to avoid chilling.
- Make sure the room temperature is cool but comfortable.
- Check for a history of febrile seizures.
- Teach the parents how to maintain a fluid intake and output record if the child is at home; if the child is hospitalized, teach the parents how to measure and record oral intake and urine output.
- Evaluate fluid intake and output totals for relative equivalency; output should be at least 1 ml/kg/hour.
- Assess skin turgor and urine specific gravity and check for fontanel depression every 4 hours.
- Obtain the child's pre-illness weight to use as the baseline. Weigh the child daily using the same clothes and scale.

NURSING DIAGNOSIS

High risk for infection (in others) related to lack of knowledge about transmission prevention

DESIRED PATIENT OUTCOME

The child will not transmit disease to others

Outcome measurement criteria

- □ Axillary temperature at or below 98° F (36.7° C); oral or tympanic temperature at or below 99° F (37.2° C)
- □ Healed, dry lesions
- □ Absence of signs of pathogen transfer to family members or others
- □ Verbalization by the parents of the need to prevent transmission
- □ Demonstration by the parents of methods to prevent transmission

Key interventions

- Teach the parents to take the child's temperature regularly and observe lesions for healing.
- Teach the parents the transmission route of the child's specific communicable disease.
- Teach the parents, caretakers, and child to prevent transmission by using correct hand-washing technique (washing hands with a specified germicide before and after every contact with the child and thoroughly washing the entire surface of each hand, including the skin between fingers); isolating the child from other children or susceptible adults; disposing of secretions in a plastic bag that has been secured at the top; having the child cover the mouth and nose when coughing or sneezing and wash hands afterward; and washing dishes and silverware with hot, soapy water (preferably in dishwasher) or using disposable utensils.
- Caution the parents to be especially careful not to expose infants, pregnant women, or chronically ill people to the child.

NURSING DIAGNOSIS

Altered comfort related to pruritus

DESIRED PATIENT OUTCOME

The child will experience partial or complete relief from pruritus

Outcome measurement criteria

- ☐ Verbalization by the parents or child that pruritus has decreased
- ☐ Absence of crying by the child
- ☐ Age-appropriate vital signs
- ☐ Absence of scratching or rubbing of lesions by the child
- ☐ Relaxed appearance and participation in play by the child

Key interventions

- Trim the child's fingernails and keep them clean.
- Place mittens or socks on the child's hands if scratching persists.
- Provide diversionary activities for the child and use positive reinforcement, such as a prize after a day of not scratching.
- Apply prescribed lotion or spray, such as calamine or topical diphenhydramine (Benadryl) spray, to affected area.
- Administer prescribed medication, such as an antipruritic agent or antihistamine.

NURSING DIAGNOSIS

Altered health maintenance related to lack of knowledge about immunization schedule

DESIRED PATIENT OUTCOME

The child will receive immunizations against childhood communicable diseases on schedule

Outcome measurement criteria

- ☐ Verbalization by the parents that the child needs to be fully immunized
- ☐ Consistent keeping of the child's immunization appointments

Key interventions

- Explain to the parents the recommended childhood immunization schedule: diphtheria, tetanus, and pertussis vaccine at ages 2, 4, 6, and 15 to 18 months and at ages 4 to 6 years or before school entry; diphtheria and tetanus booster at ages 14 to 16; oral polio virus vaccine at ages 2, 4, and 15 to 18 months and at ages 4 to 6 years or before school entry; measles, mumps, and rubella vaccine at age 15 months and at ages 11 to 12 years or before entering middle school or junior high school; *Haemophilus* b conjugate vaccine at ages 2, 4, 6, and 12 to 15 months; and hepatitis B vaccine at birth and ages 1 to 2 months and 6 to 18 months or on the schedule recommended by the vaccine manufacturer.
- Teach the parents the importance of having the child tested for tuberculosis at ages 12 to 15 months, 4 to 6 years (before school entry), and 14 to 16 years. Advise that more frequent testing may be necessary if tuberculosis is prevalent.
- Assist the parents in choosing a clinic and in arranging for transportation to it, if necessary. Provide information on clinics offering free or inexpensive vaccination services (for parents with limited incomes) and evening hours (for working parents).

Foreign body aspiration

Inhalation of an object, resulting in partial or total obstruction of a section of the airway.

NURSING DIAGNOSIS

Ineffective airway clearance related to obstruction by a foreign body

DESIRED PATIENT OUTCOME

The child will have a patent airway, free from the foreign body

Outcome measurement criteria

- ☐ Ability to move air through the larynx to speak
- ☐ Clear breath sounds in both lungs
- ☐ Symmetrical respiratory efforts
- ☐ Absence of signs of respiratory distress
- ☐ Axillary temperature below 98° F (36.7° C); tympanic temperature below 99° F (37.2° C)
- ☐ Absence of signs of infection

Key interventions

- Perform the abdominal thrust (Heimlich maneuver) if the child cannot breathe, speak, or cry.
- Obtain from the parents the history of this and similar events.
- Describe and record respiratory efforts and lung sounds.
- Assess for signs of respiratory distress, such as stridor, retractions, coughing, nasal flaring, wheezing, and tachypnea.

- Monitor for vital signs outside the normal range.
- Assess the appearance of sputum and report abnormally thick, yellow-green, or blood-tinged sputum.
- Prepare the parents and child (if age-appropriate) for foreign body removal.
- Prepare a high-humidity environment for the child after foreign body removal.
- Keep the child well hydrated.
- Avoid giving the child anything by mouth (after foreign body removal) until the gag reflex returns.
- Teach the parents respiratory therapy measures so that therapy can continue when the child returns home.
- Administer prescribed antibiotics and explain to the parents the importance of completing the entire prescription.

NURSING DIAGNOSIS

High risk for aspiration related to lack of knowledge about preventing foreign body aspiration

DESIRED PATIENT OUTCOME

The child will not aspirate a foreign body

Outcome measurement criteria

- ☐ Absence of incidents of foreign body aspiration
- ☐ Verbalization by the parents of measures to prevent aspiration
- ☐ Identification by the parents of aspiration-induced behaviors
- ☐ Demonstration of the abdominal thrust by family members

Key interventions

- Instruct the parents not to feed the young child foods that easily cause choking, such as popcorn, seeds, nuts, hard chips or crackers, or small pieces of vegetables, candy, or hot dogs.
- Remove small objects, such as buttons, beads, coins, balloons, and small toys, from the young child's bed and play area.
- Advise the parents that many toys are labeled with an age-group designation; instruct them to buy the child age-appropriate toys.
- Teach the parents to recognize aspiration-induced behaviors, such as coughing, gagging, stridor, wheezing, labored respirations, cyanosis, and inability to speak or cry.
- Teach the parents and school-age or older siblings how to perform the abdominal thrust.

Infectious lesions

Wounds or sores containing pathogenic microorganisms that, if transmitted, can cause disease in another person or in another location on the child.

NURSING DIAGNOSIS

High risk for infection (in others) related to lack of knowledge about the condition and its prevention

DESIRED PATIENT OUTCOME

The child will not transmit pathogens to others

Outcome measurement criteria

- ☐ Axillary temperature at or below 98° F (36.7° C); oral or tympanic temperature at or below 99° F (37.2° C)
- ☐ Healed lesions
- ☐ Absence of signs of pathogen transfer to family members and others
- ☐ Verbalization by the parents of the need to prevent disease transmission
- ☐ Demonstration by the parents and child (if age-appropriate) of methods to prevent disease transmission

Key interventions

- Instruct the parents to take the child's temperature every 4 hours or more often if needed.
- Explain to the parents that they may safely use an axillary or a tympanic thermometer for children of all ages or an oral thermometer if the child is school-age or older and can cooperate.

- Teach the parents to properly prepare, use, clean, and store the thermometer. (For details, see page 11.)
- Explain the importance of frequent hand washing to the parents and child (if age-appropriate).
- Demonstrate for the parents and other caretakers the correct hand-washing technique: wash hands with a specified germicide before taking the child's temperature and before and after contact with the child, thoroughly washing the entire surface of each hand, including areas between fingers.
- Instruct the parents that the child should sleep alone until lesions are healed.
- Teach the parents to wash and dry linens using a hot temperature setting until lesions are healed, to wash toys with a germicide and keep articles that cannot be washed from the child until lesions are healed, to prevent contact between the child and siblings unless lesions are covered, and to discard dressings from infectious lesions in plastic bags that have been secured at the top.
- Teach the parents how to clean noninfected lesions and to prevent subsequent infection of lesions.

Infectious mononucleosis

A mildly contagious, self-limiting disease that produces acute pharyngitis, malaise, fever, and enlarged lymph nodes.

NURSING DIAGNOSIS

Altered health maintenance related to lack of knowledge about mononucleosis

DESIRED PATIENT OUTCOME

The parents and child will demonstrate accurate knowledge about mononucleosis

Outcome measurement criteria

□ Verbalization of knowledge about mononucleosis

□ Demonstration of appropriate self-care during the disease, including adequate sleep and rest, appropriate nutrition, and avoidance of abdominal pressure or trauma

□ Freedom from secondary infections

□ Verbalization of comfort

Key interventions

- Assess the parents' and child's knowledge of the disease and its treatment, including bed rest, diet, and other supportive therapy, and occasional complications, such as chronic liver problems, lung and heart inflammations, and blood dyscrasias.
- Encourage a soft diet if pharyngitis occurs.

- Relieve throat discomfort by offering medication, such as acetaminophen or analgesic throat lozenges, and by encouraging warm gargles and intake of clear, warm beverages.
- Encourage a diet that has sufficient nutrients and calories to promote normal growth.
- Limit contact with people other than family members during the first few weeks of the disease to avoid secondary infection.
- Plan additional rest periods for the child, with quiet or restful distraction activities, such as reading, games, television, and movies.
- Assure the parents and child that the disease probably will not limit the child's activities for a prolonged period.
- Make the child aware of the need to avoid abdominal trauma or pressure.
- Teach the older child to check his or her temperature if it seems elevated. Advise the child that acetaminophen may be used every 4 hours for a temperature above 101° F (38.3° C).
- Encourage a follow-up visit with the primary care practitioner to detect long-term problems caused by the acute disease.

Insect infestation

Parasitic invasion of the skin or hair.

NURSING DIAGNOSIS

High risk for infection (in others) related to lack of knowledge about the condition and transmission prevention

DESIRED PATIENT OUTCOME

The child will not transmit the infestation to others

Outcome measurement criteria

- ☐ Absence of infestation in the child
- ☐ Healing of all lesions
- ☐ Age-appropriate body temperature
- ☐ Absence of signs of infestation transmission to family members
- ☐ Verbalization by the parents of the need to prevent infestation transmission
- ☐ Verbalization or demonstration, or both, by the parents of methods to prevent transmission

Key interventions

- Teach the parents the necessary child care to eliminate infestation.
- Apply pediculicide medication according to package instructions, repeating as directed.
- Use a fine-toothed comb to remove nits from hair after medication has been used to treat pediculosis.
- Have the child sleep alone until the infestation is eliminated.

- After use, soak combs and brushes in boiling water for 10 minutes.
- Wash and dry clothes and linens using the hot temperature setting until infestation is eliminated.
- Wash toys daily with a germicide; refrain from giving the child articles that cannot be washed; and vacuum carpets, upholstered furniture, and mattresses daily until the infestation is eliminated.
- Seal nonwashable articles, such as stuffed toys and pillows, in plastic for 14 days to kill insects.
- Avoid using the combs and head coverings of infested people.
- Avoid skin-to-skin contact with infested people.

NURSING DIAGNOSIS

High risk for infection (secondary) related to pruritus

DESIRED PATIENT OUTCOME

The child will display no signs of secondary infection of lesions

Outcome measurement criteria

- ☐ Healing of all lesions
- ☐ Axillary temperature below 98° F (36.7° C); oral or tympanic temperature below 99° F (37.2° C)
- ☐ Absence of pruritus

Key interventions

- Instruct the parents to administer an antihistamine as prescribed to decrease the child's pruritus.
- Teach the parents to check lesions for signs of secondary infection, such as redness and purulence.

- Teach the parents to check the child's temperature if lesions become secondarily infected.
- Teach the child correct hand-washing technique and the importance of frequent hand washing.
- Demonstrate correct hand-washing technique for the parents and other caretakers, advising them to wash hands with a specified germicide before and after contact with the child and to wash thoroughly the entire surface of each hand, including areas between fingers.
- Teach the parents about administering the prescribed antibiotic if the child's lesions become secondarily infected. Advise them to follow the instructions on the container about taking on a full or empty stomach, to provide adequate hydration, and to complete the entire course of the prescribed antibiotic. Inform the parents of adverse reactions to antibiotics and instruct them to call the primary care practitioner if reactions occur.

Poisoning, acute

Ingestion, inhalation, or absorption of a toxic substance.

NURSING DIAGNOSIS

High risk for poisoning related to insufficient parental knowledge about poisoning prevention

DESIRED PATIENT OUTCOME

The child will avoid poisoning because the parents will take appropriate defensive actions

Outcome measurement criteria

- ☐ Absence of incidents of accidental poisoning
- ☐ Verbalization by the parents of poisoning threats specific to each age-group
- ☐ Verbalization by the parents of common household hazards that can result in child poisoning
- ☐ Preventive measures in place in the home

Key interventions

- Advise the parents of situations that place children of different age-groups at risk for poisoning. Explain that infants may be given too much medication when ill or may find pills that accidentally have been dropped on the floor, that toddlers may be able to reach previously inaccessible household poisons, that preschoolers may consume too many good-tasting vitamins or ingest their parents' medicine, and that older children and adolescents may misread directions on medicine labels, misuse or intentionally overdose on nonprescription drugs, or ingest alcohol or sniff glue.

- Teach the parents of older children and adolescents to be alert for signs of substance experimentation, such as red eyes, rapid mood swings, dropping grades, isolation, antisocial behavior, and changes in friends.
- Teach the parents that the most common poisons are prescription drugs, cold preparations, acetaminophen (Tylenol), iron tablets, vitamins, house and yard plants, cleaning agents, dishwasher soap, and alcohol.
- Teach the parents safety precautions, such as placing medications, cleaning agents, and petroleum-based products in locked cabinets; putting purses containing medications in inaccessible places; discarding old batteries containing acid; suspending houseplants in inaccessible baskets; and carefully monitoring children playing near shrubs and flowers. Advise the parents never to store a substance in a container other than the original one, never to refer to medicine as candy, and to immediately seek help when older children or adolescents talk about suicide.

NURSING DIAGNOSIS

High risk for injury related to insufficient parental knowledge about first aid for accidental poisoning

DESIRED PATIENT OUTCOME

The child will receive appropriate treatment by parents if accidental poisoning occurs

Outcome measurement criteria

- ☐ Verbalization by the parents of appropriate actions to take when a child has been or is suspected to have been poisoned
- ☐ Verbalization by the parents of the importance of obtaining help immediately if accidental poisoning occurs

□ Demonstration by the parents of the correct procedure for performing cardiopulmonary resuscitation (CPR) on infants and children

□ Verbalization by the parents that emergency numbers are located beside the home telephone

□ Presence of ipecac syrup in the home

Key interventions

- Advise the parents to keep a list near the home telephone of emergency numbers for the poison control center, emergency department, pediatrician's office, and emergency response services (911).
- Teach the parents the importance of remaining calm so that they can take better actions, avoid frightening the child, and make themselves understood to emergency response dispatchers and emergency care providers.
- Teach the parents the importance of giving emergency personnel the best possible history of what has occurred.
- Instruct the parents to identify the poisoning substance and, if possible, to take a container or sample of it to the emergency department when the child is transported.
- Tell the parents to administer ipecac syrup with at least one glass of water if emergency response personnel instruct them to induce vomiting. Advise the parents that a primary care practitioner should prescribe the amount of ipecac syrup to be given to an infant; that the toddler, preschooler, or school-age child should receive 3 teaspoons (15 ml) of ipecac syrup; and that the adolescent should receive 1 oz (30 ml).
- Warn the parents *not* to induce vomiting if the poison is a caustic or corrosive substance (such as acid, disinfectant, cleaning solution, ammonia, or dishwasher soap) or a hydrocarbon or petroleum product (such as gasoline, kerosene, cleaning or lighter fluid, or paint thinner).

- Advise the parents to give water immediately to the child who has ingested a caustic or corrosive substance and to take the child to the emergency department.
- Advise the parents not to induce vomiting in the child who has ingested a hydrocarbon or petroleum product, but to take the child to the emergency department immediately.
- Warn the parents *not* to induce vomiting if the child is unconscious or drowsy.
- Instruct the parents to move the child who has inhaled a poisonous substance to a well-ventilated area.
- Advise the parents to flush the child's eye with a gentle stream of lukewarm tap water for at least 15 minutes if chemicals contact the eye and to remove the child's clothes and flush the skin with water if chemicals are on the clothing or skin.
- Instruct the parents to save any excretions, including urine, vomitus, and stool, and take them with the child to the emergency department.
- Teach the parents to administer CPR if needed to maintain breathing and heart rate.

NURSING DIAGNOSIS

Anxiety (parental) related to uncertainty about the outcome of the child's poisoning

DESIRED PATIENT OUTCOME

The parents will demonstrate an ability to cope effectively with the child's poisoning

Outcome measurement criteria

□ Verbalization by the parents of anxiety, anger, and other feelings

- ☐ Verbalization by the parents of previously successful coping techniques
- ☐ Description by the parents of increasing comfort with the situation

Key interventions

- Relate to the parents in a nonjudgmental manner.
- Encourage the parents to express anger, uncertainty about the child's condition, and other feelings.
- Update the parents frequently on the child's treatment and response to treatment.
- Have the parents discuss previous stressful parenting situations and describe how they successfully coped.
- Help the parents apply successful coping strategies.
- Encourage the parents to participate in appropriate aspects of care, such as comforting the child.
- Permit the parents to be with the child as much and as soon as possible during emergency care.

Stings and bites

Injuries to the skin caused by insects or other animals; often accompanied by venom injection or pathogen introduction into the wound.

NURSING DIAGNOSIS

Impaired tissue integrity related to stings and bites

DESIRED PATIENT OUTCOME

The child will experience only temporary tissue impairment from the sting or bite

Outcome measurement criteria

- ☐ Healed sting or bite
- ☐ Axillary temperature below 98° F (36.7° C); oral or tympanic temperature below 99° F (37.2° C)
- ☐ Absence of lasting disfigurement or long-term complications
- ☐ Completed course of antibiotic, if prescribed
- ☐ Verbal or nonverbal communication indicating relief from discomfort caused by the sting or bite

Key interventions

- Calm the child and parents.
- Instruct the parents to seek medical attention for animal and snake bites, multiple insect bites, and insect bites in a child with a known allergy to them.
- Teach the parents to identify or describe the animal, snake, or insect that inflicted the sting or bite.

- Instruct the parents to request assistance from the police or other local government agency in capturing an animal or snake, if possible. Advise them that an animal must be observed for 10 days to detect rabies and that a snake's venom can be identified more accurately if the snake is captured.
- Teach the parents to immobilize the injured area if the injury is a bite from a poisonous snake, spider, insect, or other animal and is below heart level.
- Advise the parents to take the child with a poisonous bite to the emergency department and to be prepared to give cardiopulmonary resuscitation if needed.
- Administer a tetanus, antivenin, or rabies vaccine if prescribed.
- Provide appropriate care for the child who is hospitalized. For example, monitor intravenous antibiotics if prescribed; administer analgesics as prescribed for large wounds or poisonous bites; monitor the child's vital signs; alert the primary care practitioner to impending shock, respiratory collapse, or neurologic changes; note the amount of edema hourly; and note the wound's appearance every 4 hours.
- Clean large wounds with large amounts of water; also use soap on the area surrounding a wound.
- Clean small bites with alcohol and hydrogen peroxide.
- Teach the parents to administer antihistamines and analgesics for stings; caution the parents to have emergency epinephrine available for a child with a known allergy to insect bites.
- Advise the parents to administer the full course of an oral antibiotic, if prescribed.

Sudden infant death syndrome

Unexpected, unexplained death of an apparently healthy infant, usually while the infant is sleeping.

NURSING DIAGNOSIS

Altered family processes related to an infant's death caused by sudden infant death syndrome (SIDS)

DESIRED PATIENT OUTCOME

The family will cope effectively with the infant's death

Outcome measurement criteria

- ☐ Verbalization of feelings by the parents, siblings, and other relatives
- ☐ Demonstration of mutual support by family members
- ☐ Participation by parents in a SIDS support group or visitation by parents with others who have lost an infant to SIDS
- ☐ Return of the parents to usual activities of daily living

Key interventions

- Encourage the parents, siblings, and other relatives to ask questions and express feelings.
- Encourage the parents, siblings, and other relatives to support one another.
- Provide privacy for the family after the infant is pronounced dead.
- Assist with initial procedures after death occurs, such as calling a funeral home, contacting friends and relatives, and calling a religious leader, if the parents desire.
- Allow the parents to hold the dead infant if they wish.

- Assure the parents that they or other caretakers are not at fault for the infant's death.
- Follow up with a home visit to provide current information about SIDS; talk to family members about everyday life situations, such as sleeping, eating, and returning to work or school; listen to and encourage the expression of feelings; provide information about SIDS organizations or encourage the parents to seek out other SIDS parents; and suggest counseling if coping is ineffective.

Cardiac catheterization

A diagnostic procedure in which a fluoroscope is used to pass a catheter through the blood vessels and into the heart chambers.

NURSING DIAGNOSIS

Anxiety related to lack of knowledge about the cardiac catheterization procedure and home care

DESIRED PATIENT OUTCOME

The parents and child will express reduced anxiety about cardiac catheterization and related home care

Outcome measurement criteria

- ☐ Correct statement of what will occur during and after cardiac catheterization
- ☐ Verbalization of concerns about cardiac catheterization
- ☐ Correct description of home care required for the insertion site and the involved extremity
- ☐ Verbalization of reduced anxiety about the procedure and related home care

Key interventions

- Give the parents accurate information about the risks associated with the procedure.
- Encourage the parents and child (if age-appropriate) to ask questions and discuss concerns about cardiac catheterization and possible findings; correct inaccurate information.

- Inform the parents and child about pre–cardiac catheterization testing, including electrocardiography, chest X-ray, and blood tests.
- Orient the parents to the hospital waiting room; orient the parents and child to the cardiac catheterization laboratory.
- Introduce the parents and child to the hospital staff who will work with the child.
- Allow the child (if age-appropriate) to see and play with sample instruments that will be used during cardiac catheterization.
- Give the parents and child accurate verbal and written information about cardiac catheterization. Explain that the child will be transported to the catheterization laboratory on a stretcher, may take a security object, will receive preoperative medication to relax, and will feel drowsy during the procedure. Note that the staff may play music and talk during the procedure and that the laboratory's sights and sounds will include dim lighting, a buzzing sound as X-ray films are taken, and the beeping of monitors. Also explain that the child will feel a cool sensation during preparation of the insertion site (usually in the groin area) and will feel pressure and a warm sensation when X-ray films are taken and that restraints will be placed on the arms and legs, vital signs will be monitored continuously, a pressure bandage or weight will be applied to the catheter insertion site, and the procedure will take 2 to 5 hours.
- Provide information about the immediate recovery period. Explain that the parents may be present; pressure will be applied to the insertion site, if needed; the child must remain in bed for 6 hours with the leg straight if the groin is the insertion site; and the child probably will remain sedated. Note that every 15 minutes the insertion site will be inspected for blood clots and bleeding, vital signs will be taken, and the leg

will be inspected for color, sensation, edema, temperature, pedal pulse, and capillary refill.

- Explain care that occurs after the child is awake. Note that fluids will be encouraged when the child shows no signs of nausea or vomiting and that pain will be assessed using the children's pain scale, analgesia will be provided as needed, and the pain scale will be used again 30 minutes later to assess pain relief.
- Provide information to the parents and child about home care. Advise the parents to wash their hands before inspecting the insertion site; to inspect the site daily for drainage, redness, swelling, and bleeding; and to inspect the extremity distal to the insertion site at least twice daily for color, sensation, mobility, swelling, and temperature. Also instruct them to take the child's temperature twice daily, to administer prophylactic antibiotics as prescribed, and to report to the primary care practitioner fever, extensive pain, or problems with the insertion site or extremity.
- Give the parents a telephone number to call if questions or problems arise.

NURSING DIAGNOSIS

High risk for infection related to wound and cardiac catheterization

DESIRED PATIENT OUTCOME

The child will remain free from infection

Outcome measurement criteria

☐ Axillary temperature below 99° F (37.2° C) for the first 2 days after the procedure and at or below 98° F (36.7° C) thereafter; oral or tympanic temperature below 100° F (37.8° C) for the first 2 days after the procedure and at or below 99° F (37.2° C) thereafter

- ☐ Pink incision and other wound sites; absence of purulence
- ☐ Absence of chest pain
- ☐ Responsiveness and alertness of the child
- ☐ Demonstration by the parents of the correct technique for taking the child's temperature
- ☐ Verbalization by the parents of the need to call the primary care practitioner if signs of infection occur
- ☐ Absence of pain in the affected extremity

Key interventions

- Monitor the child's temperature. Expect a low fever for the first few days after the procedure; a high fever may indicate a systemic infection or a localized infection of the heart or chest.
- Assess other vital signs every 4 hours after the immediate recovery period; check more frequently if complications arise.
- Administer prescribed prophylactic antibiotics beginning the day before the procedure and continuing for 4 to 5 days afterward.
- Monitor for increased number of leukocytes and elevated sedimentation rate.
- Monitor urine specific gravity, which should range from 1.010 to 1.025.
- Monitor fluid intake and output.
- Examine mucous membranes for moistness.
- Examine skin turgor for elasticity.
- Examine the anterior fontanel (if patent) to ensure that it is flat—not depressed or bulging.
- Teach the parents to recognize the signs and symptoms of infection at home, such as fever and malaise.

Congestive heart failure

Inability of the heart to pump sufficient blood to meet the child's needs, usually caused by congenital heart defects in an infant or a young child.

NURSING DIAGNOSIS

Activity intolerance related to insufficient oxygen supply secondary to congestive heart failure (CHF)

DESIRED PATIENT OUTCOME

The child will demonstrate reduced cardiac demand and oxygen consumption

Outcome measurement criteria

- ☐ Age-appropriate vital signs
- ☐ Absence of dyspnea
- ☐ Pulse oximetry reading appropriate to the cardiac defect present and the amount of repair completed
- ☐ Absence of signs of infection
- ☐ Axillary temperature at or below 98° F (36.7° C); oral or tympanic temperature at or below 99° F (37.2° C)
- ☐ Tolerance of oral feeding
- ☐ Weight within normal range
- ☐ Calm, peaceful demeanor

Key interventions

- Take vital signs every hour initially and then every 4 hours, counting the apical pulse for 1 full minute.
- Monitor serum electrolyte levels.

- Place the child in semi-Fowler's position in an infant seat or cardiac chair; elevate the head of the bed for an older child.
- Suction the airway to maintain patency; deliver additional oxygen immediately before and after suctioning.
- Administer oxygen with humidity using an oxygen hood or a tent; use a mask or nasal cannula on an older child who can tolerate it.
- Monitor the blood oxygen level using pulse oximetry.
- Monitor for signs of infection, such as an increased temperature.
- Administer antibiotics if infection is present.
- Administer heart and other medications accurately as prescribed and monitor the child for adverse reactions.
- Strictly maintain fluid intake and output records; urine output must be at least 1 ml/kg/hour.
- Check that urine specific gravity falls within the age-appropriate range.
- Restrict fluids to 1,000 ml/m^2/day, if prescribed.
- Administer parenteral fluids until the child can tolerate oral feedings without excessive dyspnea. Then give small oral feedings every 2 hours.
- Weigh the child every shift during the acute phase, using the same scale and same clothing. Thereafter, weigh the child daily.
- Keep the infant calm and comforted by giving a pacifier, rocking, or stroking; provide the older child with quiet, restful activities.
- Cluster care activities to allow the child maximum rest.
- Encourage the parents to participate in the child's care as much as possible.

NURSING DIAGNOSIS

High risk for ineffective management of therapeutic regimen (parental) related to the complexity of the regimen to treat CHF

DESIRED PATIENT OUTCOME

The parents will manage the child's care effectively after discharge

Outcome measurement criteria

- ☐ Verbalization by the parents of accurate knowledge about the child's condition
- ☐ Verbalization by the parents of the child's required care at home
- ☐ Demonstration by the parents of correct vital sign measurement, including apical pulse palpation
- ☐ Demonstration by the parents of administration of digoxin and other medications as prescribed
- ☐ Consistent keeping by the parents of the child's clinic or office appointments
- ☐ Verbalization by the parents of comfort with caring for the child at home

Key interventions

- Teach the parents how to recognize the signs and symptoms of CHF: lethargy, fatigue while eating, poor weight gain, increased pulse and breathing rates, sweating, costal retractions, and nasal flaring.
- Teach the parents how to take the apical pulse before administering each digoxin dose. Demonstrate and then have the parents demonstrate correct measurement of medication and apical pulse rate. Tell the parents to administer the dose to an infant very slowly into the side of the mouth to prevent choking.

- Instruct the parents to administer digoxin according to the prescribed schedule when the child's stomach is empty and not to mix food with digoxin.
- Advise the parents not to miss a dose, to wait until the next regularly scheduled time if a dose is delayed more than 4 hours, to give a missed dose if it is delayed less than 4 hours, to call the primary care practitioner if more than two consecutive doses are missed, and never to increase or double a dose.
- Instruct the parents to notify the primary care practitioner and not repeat the dose if the child vomits or becomes ill or if the pulse rate is below 90 beats/minute in an infant or a young child or below 70 beats/minute in a school-age child.
- Advise the parents to lock the cabinet containing digoxin.
- Teach the parents of the child taking a diuretic to administer it early in the day, to monitor for weight changes, and to monitor for signs of low potassium levels, such as weakness, orthostatic hypotension, muscle cramps, vomiting, fatigue, drowsiness, confusion, and bradycardia.
- Advise the parents to give potassium-rich foods (such as bananas, oranges, and whole grains) or prescribed potassium supplements in juice (to disguise the taste and prevent stomach irritation) and then to monitor for signs of high potassium levels, such as confusion, weakness, hyperexcitability, twitching, GI upset, and arrhythmias.
- Advise parents of the importance of keeping clinic or office appointments.
- Encourage the parents to ask questions and express feelings.

Heart defects, congenital

Cardiac anomalies present at birth that produce varying degrees of limitation.

NURSING DIAGNOSIS

Anxiety related to lack of knowledge about surgery for congenital heart defects

DESIRED PATIENT OUTCOME

The parents and child will verbalize reduced anxiety about corrective surgery

Outcome measurement criteria

- ☐ Verbalization by the parents and child (if age-appropriate) of the need for surgery to correct heart defects
- ☐ Description by the parents and child (if age-appropriate) of the requirements and anticipated outcomes of surgery
- ☐ Verbalization by the parents and child (if age-appropriate) of expectations during postoperative intensive care
- ☐ Statement by the parents and child (if age-appropriate) that their concerns are now more manageable

Key interventions

- Clarify with the primary care practitioner what information has been given to the parents and child.
- Explain the child's heart defects to the parents verbally and pictorially. For example, show a videotape and then answer questions.
- Inform the parents why surgery is needed.

- Discuss with the parents the anticipated outcomes and how they will improve the child's and family's lives.
- Orient the child and parents to the cardiac unit and intensive care unit (ICU).
- Allow the child to touch selected equipment and hear sounds that will occur in the cardiac unit and ICU.
- Show the child how the hospital staff will look when wearing masks, gowns, and goggles or shields.
- Demonstrate surgery, bandaging, and treatments to the child, using puppets or dolls.
- Explain to the parents and child the treatments and tubes (I.V., urinary catheter, oxygen, nasogastric) that will be used, and discuss the reasons for each.
- Explain to the parents and child that preoperative medication will be given and will cause drowsiness.
- Explain that the child will be asleep during surgery. Provide reassurance that the child will not awaken until afterward.
- Demonstrate to the parents how the ventilator works, and explain how it will help the child.
- Show the parents where they can wait during surgery.
- Explain to the parents the visiting policies in various pediatric units.
- Tell the parents the approximate number of days the child will be hospitalized.
- Explain to the parents and child that medications will be given to enhance comfort after surgery. Also explain the use of the children's pain scale.
- Encourage the parents to visit with other parents whose children have had similar surgery.

NURSING DIAGNOSIS

Anxiety related to the unknown outcome of surgery for congenital heart defects

DESIRED PATIENT OUTCOME

The parents will demonstrate reduced anxiety related to corrective surgery

Outcome measurement criteria

- ☐ Verbalization by the parents to each other and the hospital staff of their fears
- ☐ Accurate verbalization by the parents of the child's reported condition and progress
- ☐ Verbalization by the parents of increased comfort with the ICU atmosphere and the hospital environment
- ☐ Participation by the parents in the child's care, such as assisting in feeding, bathing, and comforting
- ☐ Demonstration by the parents of mutual support, such as standing close together, communicating openly, or touching or holding each other

Key interventions

- Orient the parents to the ICU before surgery.
- Reorient the parents when the child arrives in the ICU and the pediatric unit.
- Encourage the parents to openly discuss with each other their feelings and fears.
- Encourage the parents to initiate discussions with the staff about feelings and fears.
- Frequently provide the parents with accurate information on the child's condition.
- Allow the parents to stay with the child as much as possible.

- As soon as possible after surgery, review with the parents the treatments and use of tubes.
- Encourage the parents and child to participate actively in care, as appropriate.
- Encourage the parents to be involved in decision making about the child's care.
- Encourage the parents to talk with, stroke, and hold the child, if possible, and encourage family members to read stories or sing to the child.
- Provide support for the child to express feelings through play activities, such as drawing, hammering pegs, pounding clay, squeezing toys, and playing age-appropriate games.
- Give the toddler or older child choices about care, such as who will bathe the child and assist with walking and which of two equally appropriate foods and sequences of medicines to take.

NURSING DIAGNOSIS

Ineffective breathing pattern related to the effects of surgery for congenital heart defects

DESIRED PATIENT OUTCOME

The child will display an effective breathing pattern

Outcome measurement criteria

☐ Chest tube drainage not to exceed 2 ml/kg/hour

☐ Evidence of lung reinflation on chest X-ray

☐ Vital signs within age-appropriate ranges

☐ Clear, symmetrical breath sounds

☐ Pulse oximetry reading appropriate to the cardiac problem and the amount of repair completed

☐ Normal cardiac rhythm (if repair is complete)

Key interventions

- Explain all procedures and treatments to the parents and child.
- Check the chest drainage equipment to ensure that the drainage tube is straight, tubing connections are taped, the dressing is secured over the chest entry site, and the drainage system unit is well secured below the child's chest level.
- For each chest tube, keep two clamps available, adjacent to the water seal setup, for emergency use.
- Measure chest tube drainage by marking the level and time on the collection chamber every 15 minutes immediately after surgery, every hour for the next 24 hours, and every 4 hours thereafter, unless otherwise indicated.
- Record the color of chest tube drainage. Notify the physician if bloody drainage equals or exceeds 3 ml/kg for 3 hours.
- Check chest tubes for patency.
- Report to the physician any of the following: dyspnea, sudden changes in breath sounds or lack of breath sounds on the affected side, hyperresonance of chest on percussion, or absence of chest tube drainage even though chest tubes are patent.
- Premedicate the child 30 minutes before chest tube removal.
- Tell the child to expect sharp pain during chest tube removal but that it will not last long.
- Assist with chest X-rays.
- Monitor ventilator functioning and the child's response to it.

- Suction the child every 1 to 2 hours and as needed. Remember to hyperoxygenate before and after suctioning, use sterile technique, and use suction (negative pressure) only after positioning the catheter in the appropriate part of the respiratory tract.
- Monitor for respiratory distress after extubation.
- Turn the child and have the child breathe deeply. Splint the chest with pillows.
- Give pain medication 30 to 40 minutes before chest physiotherapy.
- Ensure that chest physiotherapy is completed on time. Note the effects of treatments.
- Monitor vital signs for indications of inadequate oxygenation.
- Report cyanosis or restlessness.
- Assess cardiac activity via a monitor.
- Auscultate and percuss lung fields each time vital signs are taken.
- Inspect the chest for bilateral symmetry of movements.
- Help the child walk on the 2nd or 3rd postoperative day, if possible.
- Encourage the parents to participate in some aspects of care, such as comforting and turning the child.

NURSING DIAGNOSIS

Fluid volume deficit related to surgery for congenital heart defects

DESIRED PATIENT OUTCOME

The child will display adequate fluid volume

Outcome measurement criteria

- ☐ Elastic skin turgor
- ☐ Flat fontanel (if patent)
- ☐ Warm arms and legs
- ☐ Age-appropriate vital signs
- ☐ Strong and equal peripheral pulses
- ☐ Capillary refill time of less than 2 seconds
- ☐ Normal cardiac rhythm
- ☐ Dressing with minimal drainage
- ☐ Urine output of at least 1 ml/kg/hour
- ☐ Electrolyte and blood gas levels within normal ranges
- ☐ Age-appropriate urine specific gravity
- ☐ Moist mucous membranes
- ☐ Age-appropriate fluid intake and output

Key interventions

- Monitor the I.V. infusion site and fluids; ensure that the prescribed amount is infused on time.
- Strictly monitor fluid intake and output. Check urine output every hour, making sure it is at least 1 ml/kg/hour. Also check urine specific gravity every hour.
- Check the surgical dressing for drainage.
- Measure nasogastric drainage every 8 hours.
- Monitor vital signs for indications of internal bleeding.
- Assess peripheral pulses, which should be strong and equal.
- Assess the arms and legs for skin temperature and the nails for capillary refill.
- Monitor arterial blood gases.

- Monitor indwelling vascular lines, such as central venous, pulmonary artery, right atrial, and arterial pressure lines.
- Monitor serum levels of electrolytes, especially potassium.
- Administer cardiac medications as prescribed. Assess their effects on cardiac rhythm and systemic circulation and observe for adverse reactions, such as bradycardia and vomiting.
- Assess cardiac activity via a monitor.
- Observe the skin for petechiae and ecchymoses.
- Begin feeding as prescribed after bowel sounds resume. Start with ice chips or sips of water, increase to clear liquids, and then proceed to a high-carbohydrate, high-protein diet.
- Encourage the parents to participate in some aspects of care, such as feeding and bathing.

NURSING DIAGNOSIS

Pain related to tissue trauma secondary to chest surgery and hospitalization

DESIRED PATIENT OUTCOME

The child will report or display signs of an acceptable comfort level

Outcome measurement criteria

- ☐ Verbalization by the child and parents of feelings about painful procedures and treatments
- ☐ Verbalization by the child of increased comfort
- ☐ Demonstration by the child of increased comfort, such as smiling, talking, and playing

- ☐ Demonstration on the age-appropriate children's pain scale of increased comfort
- ☐ Choices by the child of measures that increase comfort

Key interventions

- Ask the parents about the child's typical reaction to pain and what usually relieves it effectively.
- Anticipate pain and offer pain-relief measures 30 minutes before painful procedures.
- Involve the parents in pain-relief measures, if possible.
- Locate the site of pain in the preschooler or older child by asking him or her to point to it.
- Assess the initial pain level using the age-appropriate children's pain scale.
- Encourage the child to tell the caregiver which measures decrease pain and increase comfort.
- Teach the child nonpharmacologic pain-relief measures, such as controlled breathing, distraction games, heat or cold, imagery, massage, music, pressure, relaxation techniques, and repositioning.
- Administer analgesics and determine their effect on pain 30 minutes after administration, using the age-appropriate children's pain scale.
- Determine the most effective pain-relief measures for common painful procedures and treatments and design a pain-relief protocol for them.
- Encourage the child and family members to express feelings about painful procedures.
- Provide opportunities for the child to play out painful experiences using dolls or hand puppets.
- Be truthful with the child about painful treatments and procedures, indicating approximately how much pain to expect and how long it will last.

- Provide privacy during and after procedures and treatments to let the child regain composure.
- Allow the parents to be present during procedures and treatments, if hospital policy permits and the parents wish.
- Encourage the child to remain still during the procedure and assure the child that it is acceptable to express pain, cry, yell, and squeeze the nurse's hand during painful procedures.
- Praise the child for enduring painful experiences.
- Encourage the parents to hold and comfort the child after a painful procedure or treatment.
- Give the child opportunities for rest and uninterrupted sleep after painful experiences.

NURSING DIAGNOSIS

Ineffective management of therapeutic regimen (parental) related to the complexity of the regimen after surgical repair of congenital heart defects

DESIRED PATIENT OUTCOME

The parents will manage care effectively after the child is discharged

Outcome measurement criteria

- ☐ Verbalization by the parents of knowledge about the child's heart defects and surgical repair
- ☐ Verbalization by the parents of the care the child will need at home
- ☐ Demonstration by the parents of how to accurately take vital signs, including the apical pulse
- ☐ Demonstration by the parents of how to administer digoxin

- ☐ Verbalization by the parents of appropriate play activities
- ☐ Consistent keeping by the parents of the child's clinic or office appointments

Key interventions

- Make all explanations consistent with the parents' educational level.
- Visually and verbally review with the parents the child's heart defects and surgical repair.
- Encourage the parents to ask questions and discuss fears.
- Teach the parents appropriate home care procedures, including how to accurately take vital signs, including apical pulse; administer digoxin as prescribed; observe the child for fatigue, irritability, shortness of breath, edema, pallor, and mottled or cyanotic appearance; assess fluid and nutritional intake and weekly weight changes; report cough or dyspnea to the primary care practitioner; allow for rest periods when feeding; provide for rest and sleep; hold or comfort the child to reduce stress; notify the primary care practitioner if the child's temperature is elevated; and protect the child from infections by washing hands and avoiding contact with crowds and infectious people.
- Teach the parents appropriate play activities.
- Emphasize the importance of keeping appointments to evaluate the child's physical and developmental status.

NURSING DIAGNOSIS

Altered family processes related to the requirements of caring for a child with congenital heart defects

DESIRED PATIENT OUTCOME

The family will adjust effectively to caring for the child with congenital heart defects

Outcome measurement criteria

- ☐ Demonstration of family members' affection by holding, touching, and warmly interacting with the child
- ☐ Open expression of feelings by the parents and siblings
- ☐ Open and appropriate communication among family members
- ☐ Demonstration by each family member of mutual support
- ☐ Accomplishment of developmental milestones by the child
- ☐ Use by the parents of community support systems to meet the family's and child's needs
- ☐ Participation by the family in the child's care
- ☐ Fulfillment by the parents of the child's health care needs
- ☐ Identification by the parents of specific factors that cause stress for the family and of appropriate responses
- ☐ Verbalization by the parents of gaining increased control of the situation

Key interventions

- Assess the family's strengths and weaknesses.
- Assess the child's physical needs and developmental status.
- Encourage family members to openly discuss their feelings.

- Explore the family's feelings of guilt, anger, sadness, and hopelessness. Offer ways to deal with these feelings, such as using coping strategies that have been used successfully in previous family crises.
- Assist the family with problem solving.
- Encourage the parents to join a support group.
- Have the family plan care for the child and divide responsibilities.
- Identify aspects of the child's illness that cause stress for individual family members, such as the need for constant care, special services, medications, additional surgery, and long-term treatment; long-term financial demands; the reactions of siblings and friends to the child's illness; decreased social interactions for family members; difficulty in obtaining a baby-sitter; and too little time for the parents as a couple or as individuals.
- Develop a plan to minimize stress-related negative reactions and behaviors by family members. For example, help the family plan time for each child in the family (the child and siblings) to receive special attention from a parent each week, plan personal time for the parents each week, and obtain respite care for the child so the parents can cultivate their relationship.

Rheumatic fever, acute

An autoimmune disease that occurs in response to a group A beta-hemolytic streptococcal infection.

NURSING DIAGNOSIS

Anxiety related to lack of knowledge about acute rheumatic fever (ARF) and its treatment

DESIRED PATIENT OUTCOME

The parents and child will demonstrate reduced anxiety about the child's disease and care

Outcome measurement criteria

- ☐ Verbalization by the parents and child of the role of a streptococcal infection in the development of ARF
- ☐ Verbalization by the parents and child of knowledge about major manifestations of ARF and care related to these manifestations
- ☐ Verbalization by the parents and child of reduced anxiety based on knowledge about the disease and its treatment

Key interventions

- Obtain a history of recent infections and related treatments.
- Inform the parents and child about the need to eradicate the streptococcal infection with antibiotics. Explain that the child will receive penicillin or erythromycin if allergic to penicillin.
- Explain to the parents and child the need for numerous laboratory tests, and discuss their role in diagnosis.

- Inform the parents about major manifestations of ARF, including polyarthritis, carditis, chorea, erythema marginatum, and subcutaneous nodules. Advise them that all major manifestations, except perhaps carditis, are temporary.
- Explain to the parents and child the care related to polyarthritis: salicylates for pain (given with meals), warm compresses applied to affected joints, bed cradle to minimize the pressure of linens on joints, minimal handling, and positioning with blanket rolls or pillows.
- Explain that care for chorea includes administering prescribed medication to decrease random movements; preventing injury from falls by using bed rails, securing the child when in a chair, and padding nearby objects; assisting with ambulation (the child cannot ambulate alone if chorea has been present recently); assisting with feeding and other self-care activities; and informing those who have contact with the child that symptoms are temporary.
- Explain that care for cardiac involvement includes administering digoxin to improve cardiac output, checking that apical pulse is over 90 beats/minute in a young child and over 70 beats/minute in a school-age child before digoxin administration, and reporting to the primary care practitioner if the pulse rate is too slow.
- Explain that care also includes administering parenteral fluids until the child can tolerate oral feedings without excessive dyspnea; using semi-Fowler's position; administering oxygen with humidity via nasal cannula; strictly recording fluid intake and output; restricting fluids to no more than 1,000 ml/m^2/day; checking urine output to ensure it is at least 1 ml/kg/hour; checking to ensure that urine specific gravity is within the age-appropriate range; weighing the child in the acute phase during every shift with the same scale and same clothing; weighing the child daily after the acute phase; checking

vital signs every hour initially and then every 4 hours and counting the apical pulse for 1 full minute; promoting calmness and comfort to reduce stress on the heart; and planning care to promote maximum rest.

- Show the parents pictures of erythema marginatum and subcutaneous nodules if the child has not yet had these manifestations.
- Explain that erythema marginatum and subcutaneous nodules are transient and require no specific care.

NURSING DIAGNOSIS

High risk for caregiver role strain related to lack of knowledge about ARF and the stress of caring for the child

DESIRED PATIENT OUTCOME

The parents and child will implement home care successfully

Outcome measurement criteria

- ☐ Description by the parents of realistic problems they will face in caring for the child at home
- ☐ Verbalization by the parents of ways to overcome these problems
- ☐ Verbalization by the parents of the information needed for successful care
- ☐ Use by the parents of recommended community and family resources
- ☐ Verbalization by the parents of feelings about care
- ☐ Statement by the parents of satisfaction with the resolution of home care problems
- ☐ Maintenance of a prophylactic antibiotic regimen for the child through young adulthood or longer

- □ Maintenance of a limited activity regimen until the erythrocyte sedimentation rate (ESR) is within normal limits for a child with no cardiac involvement, and limited activity for 1 to 2 weeks after ESR is within normal limits for a child with cardiac involvement
- □ Accurate description of possible long-term effects of rheumatic fever

Key interventions

- Teach the parents, child, and other family members about medication administration.
- Explain why long-term antibiotic therapy is needed.
- Administer prophylactic antibiotics as prescribed: oral penicillin (or erythromycin) daily or an injection of long-lasting penicillin every 3 to 4 weeks.
- Praise the child for cooperating with the medication regimen, using positive reinforcement such as rewards for compliance.
- Allow the child to be responsible for keeping a record of the date and time oral medication was administered.
- Continue antibiotic therapy until the child becomes a young adult or longer if the young adult lives with young children.
- Administer prophylactic antibiotics before dental work and other invasive procedures.
- Administer salicylates for the prescribed length of time, which varies with the severity of the disease.
- Schedule the child's appointment with the primary care practitioner to monitor the need for more salicylates.
- Record the child's complaints of pain after discontinuing salicylates. Note pain severity and location and use the age-appropriate children's pain scale. Report pain to the primary care practitioner.

- Administer a prescribed corticosteroid in gradually tapering doses (usually for 3 to 4 weeks, unless significant cardiac involvement exists). Emphasize that doses must not be skipped and that the drug must not be stopped abruptly because severe hypotension, shock, coma, or death could result.
- Report to the primary care practitioner recurring pain after steroid therapy is discontinued.
- Explain to the child why activities must be limited. Realize that preschoolers and school-age children may feel threatened by this limitation.
- Teach the parents about educational activities and diversions for the child with cardiac involvement who feels well but must limit activity. Discuss homework assignments and a home tutor; passive range-of-motion exercises; and age-appropriate activities, such as watching children's movies and television programs, listening to music and stories on tape, reading, coloring, drawing, modeling with clay, playing with dolls, writing letters, and playing cards or electronic games.
- Designate several places for the child to rest, such as a bed, beanbag chair, pallet, recliner, sofa, or lawn chair, so that the child will not become frustrated by the need to rest frequently. Mutually agree with the child on the amount of time he or she must stay in one place to rest.
- Develop a mobile activities kit by placing books, movies, music tapes, clay, pens, paper, glue, and other items into a movable object, such as a rolling television cart, rolling chair, child's toy grocery cart, or picnic basket.
- Make a list of acceptable activities, such as self-feeding, washing face and hands, and walking to the bathroom, dining table, or yard.
- Plan to take the child outside once or twice a day to sit in a chair (weather permitting).
- Reward the child for cooperation by allowing extra time outside or another activity the child values.

- Teach the parents to avoid the complications of activity restriction by allowing the child certain choices, such as a choice of eating place, game, or movie; serving frequent, small, nutritious meals that include high-fiber foods; having the child drink at least four glasses of fluid daily; and weighing the child daily, recording the weight, and presenting a weight record when visiting the primary care practitioner's office.
- Instruct the child on correct hand-washing technique and the importance of frequent hand washing.
- Teach the parents to protect the child from infections by washing their hands before and after contact with the child; not allowing the child to visit people who are ill; screening out visitors with infections; avoiding crowds when respiratory tract infections are prevalent; providing a bed in which the child can sleep alone; informing the dentist, surgeon, and other health care providers that the child has had rheumatic fever; and requiring the child to become increasingly responsible for self-care, including making decisions about protection from infections.
- Discuss with the parents the need for assistance from the extended family, community, or both with caregiving, transportation, respite care, and related activities.
- Discuss problems with implementing care at home, such as the strains of caregiving if both parents work, the cost of medication, and the difficulty in arranging follow-up visits, including transportation.
- Discuss the possibility of a recurrence of rheumatic fever and carditis and the need to comply with antibiotic therapy and avoid infections.

Chronic illness or impairment

A disease or disorder that is present at birth or develops over time and persists, often for the remainder of the child's life.

NURSING DIAGNOSIS

Anticipatory grieving related to loss of the child's health

DESIRED PATIENT OUTCOME

The parents will cope effectively with their grief at the loss of the child's health

Outcome measurement criteria

- ☐ Expression of grief by the parents
- ☐ Verbalization by the parents that reflects an understanding of grieving
- ☐ Demonstration of mutual support by family members
- ☐ Verbalization by the parents of a plan to deal with the immediate details of caring for their child

Key interventions

- Assess the parents' past experiences with grief and loss.
- Explain that grief is normal, clarify the stages of grief, and correct misconceptions.
- Identify the strengths of the family as a unit and as individuals.
- Encourage discussion by the parents of feelings about the loss of the child's health.

- Encourage the parents to be open and truthful with other family members, including the child.
- Prepare the parents for the possible responses of people to the child's condition.
- Discuss ways for the parents to handle the immediate details of care, such as providing adequate care for the child and siblings; making special arrangements with employers, as needed; making financial arrangements for child care; and modifying the home environment, as needed.

NURSING DIAGNOSIS

Anxiety related to lack of knowledge about the child's newly diagnosed illness or condition

DESIRED PATIENT OUTCOME

The child and family will demonstrate reduced anxiety and become more familiar with the illness or condition

Outcome measurement criteria

- ☐ Verbalization by the parents of accurate knowledge about the illness or condition
- ☐ Verbalization by the parents of the effects of the illness or condition on the child and family as a unit and as individuals
- ☐ Use by the parents of community support systems for learning about the illness or condition
- ☐ Participation by the family and child (if age-appropriate) in the child's care
- ☐ Return of the child and family members to usual eating and sleeping patterns
- ☐ Resumption by the family members of appropriate developmental tasks
- ☐ Resumption of play by the child and siblings

- ☐ Continued child growth and development to the degree the illness or condition permits
- ☐ Verbalization by the child (if age-appropriate) and family members of increased comfort with the newly diagnosed illness or condition
- ☐ Involvement of the family in a support group

Key interventions

- Assess the parents' and child's knowledge about the illness or condition.
- Teach the family and child about the specific illness or condition.
- Obtain a thorough history of the child's and family's experiences with hospitalization.
- Orient the parents and child to the hospital's personnel and routine.
- Encourage the child and siblings to use play to act out anxiety and fear.
- Encourage open communication among the family members and between the nurse and family members.
- Explain all procedures and tests before they are performed.
- Allow the parents to be with the child as much as possible.
- Encourage discussions by the family and child about the effects of the condition on their lifestyle.
- Plan how the child and each family member can contribute to the child's care.
- Demonstrate special care needed by the child.
- Support and provide positive feedback to the family and child as they learn aspects of care.
- Encourage the family to become involved with a support group.

- Evaluate the family's resumption of usual activities of daily living.

NURSING DIAGNOSIS

High risk for caregiver role strain related to the requirements of caring for a chronically ill or impaired child

DESIRED PATIENT OUTCOME

The family will adjust effectively to caring for the chronically ill or impaired child

Outcome measurement criteria

- ☐ Demonstration by the family members of affection for the child through holding, touching, and warm interactions
- ☐ Open expression of feelings by the parents and siblings
- ☐ Open and appropriate communication among family members
- ☐ Demonstration by each family member of mutual support
- ☐ Verbalization by the parents of achievement of normal growth and developmental milestones for the child
- ☐ Achievement of developmental milestones (modified if necessary) and appropriate social development by the child
- ☐ Use by the parents of specific community support systems to help meet the family's and child's needs
- ☐ Participation by the family in the child's care
- ☐ Fulfillment by the family of the child's health care needs
- ☐ Identification by the parents of specific factors that cause stress
- ☐ Implementation by the parents of a plan to counter the stresses of having a chronically ill child in the family

- ☐ Verbalization by the parents of gaining more control of the situation

Key interventions

- Assess the family's strengths and weaknesses.
- Assess the child's physical needs and developmental status.
- Encourage family members to discuss feelings openly.
- Explore the family's feelings of guilt, anger, sadness, and hopelessness and suggest ways to deal with these feelings.
- Encourage the parents to join a support group.
- Have the family plan care for the child and divide responsibilities.
- Identify coping strategies that family members have used successfully in previous family crises.
- Identify stressful aspects of having a chronically ill child in the family, such as the child's need for constant care, special services and medications, long-term treatment outside the home, and special schooling; long-term financial demands; reactions of siblings and siblings' friends; decreased social opportunities for family members; difficulty in obtaining a baby-sitter; too little time for the parents as a couple and as individuals; and anxiety about the child's long-term care.
- Develop a plan to minimize stress-related problems in family members. Help the parents plan time for the child and each sibling to receive special attention each week, encourage parents to provide the child with limits similar to those imposed on siblings, and help the parents obtain respite care for the child so they can cultivate their relationship as a couple and have some personal time each week.

NURSING DIAGNOSIS

Feeding, bathing, hygiene, dressing, grooming, and toileting self-care deficits related to developmental delays secondary to chronic illness or impairment

DESIRED PATIENT OUTCOME

The child and parents will adapt to meeting the child's self-care needs

Outcome measurement criteria

- ☐ Verbalization by the parents and child of feelings about the child's self-care limitations
- ☐ Demonstration by the parents and child of competence in meeting the child's self-care needs
- ☐ Verbalization by the parents and child of positive feelings about adapting to the child's self-care needs
- ☐ Use of a team of health care professionals to help meet the child's self-care needs
- ☐ Use of community resources to help meet the child's self-care needs
- ☐ Demonstration by the parents of the ability to use assistive devices

Key interventions

- Encourage the family and child to discuss feelings about the child's inability to meet self-care needs.
- Assemble a health care team to help the family and child meet the child's self-care needs.
- Demonstrate alternative ways to meet the child's self-care needs.
- Encourage the family to allow the child to assist with self-care.
- Teach the parents how to use various assistive devices.

- Assist the family in using community support systems to help meet the child's self-care needs.
- Discuss ways to obtain financial assistance to meet the child's special needs.
- Encourage the family to meet with other families in similar circumstances.

NURSING DIAGNOSIS

Altered growth and development related to frequent hospitalizations or treatments

DESIRED PATIENT OUTCOME

The child will display growth and development that, as much as possible, meets age-appropriate norms

Outcome measurement criteria

- ☐ Verbalization by the parents of age-appropriate growth and developmental norms for the child and ways to help the child to meet those norms
- ☐ Documentation by the parents of the child's weight and height gains according to age-appropriate growth norms
- ☐ Age-appropriate psychosocial, speech, motor, and intellectual development by the child
- ☐ Participation by the child in age-appropriate play
- ☐ Use by the family of community resources to enhance the child's growth and development

Key interventions

- Assess the child's current psychosocial, speech, motor, and intellectual development.
- Assess the child's nutritional status and eating patterns.

- Provide the parents with age-appropriate growth and developmental norms for the child. Instruct the parents to document growth on a monthly basis and bring charts with them to follow-up visits.
- Discuss play materials and activities to enhance the child's growth and development.
- Discuss age-appropriate nutrition needs for the child, including protein, carbohydrate, fat, vitamin, fiber, and caloric needs.
- Arrange contacts with community agencies that can offer the family support.
- Discuss activities or events that may precipitate hospitalization, such as noncompliance, pollen season, and excessive fatigue, and devise ways to curtail these activities or deal with these events.

NURSING DIAGNOSIS

Pain related to treatments or procedures for or progression of a chronic illness or impairment

DESIRED PATIENT OUTCOME

The child will report (or demonstrate) and maintain an acceptable comfort level

Outcome measurement criteria

- ☐ Verbalization by the child and parents of feelings about painful procedures and treatments
- ☐ Verbalization by the child (if age-appropriate) of increased comfort
- ☐ Demonstration by the child of increased comfort through smiling, talking, and playing
- ☐ Demonstration on the age-appropriate children's pain scale of increased comfort
- ☐ Use of measures by the child that increase comfort

Key interventions

- Anticipate pain and offer pain-relief measures 30 minutes before painful procedures.
- Ask the parents about the child's usual reaction to pain and effective relief measures.
- Involve the parents in pain-relief measures, if possible.
- Locate the site of pain in the preschooler or older child by asking him or her to point to it.
- Assess the initial pain level using the age-appropriate children's pain scale.
- Ask the child to tell the caregiver which measures decrease pain and increase comfort.
- Teach the child nonpharmacologic pain-relief measures that may be used, such as controlled breathing, distraction games, heat or cold application, imagery, massage, music, pressure, relaxation techniques, and repositioning.
- Administer analgesics and determine their effect on pain 30 minutes after administration, using the age-appropriate children's pain scale.
- Determine the most effective pain-relief measures for the painful procedures and treatments the child will undergo, and design a pain-relief protocol for them.
- Encourage the child and family to express feelings about painful procedures.
- Provide opportunities for the child to handle equipment and play out painful experiences using dolls or hand puppets.
- Be truthful with the child about painful treatments and procedures, indicating approximately how much pain will occur and how long it will last.
- Provide privacy during and after procedures and treatments to allow the child to regain composure.

- Have the parents stay with the child during procedures and treatments if hospital policy permits and parents wish.
- Encourage the child to remain still during procedures, but assure the child that it is all right to express pain, cry, yell, and squeeze the nurse's hand during painful procedures.
- Praise the child for enduring painful experiences.
- Encourage the parents to hold and comfort the child immediately after painful procedures or treatments.
- Give the child opportunities for rest and uninterrupted sleep after painful experiences.

NURSING DIAGNOSIS

Chronic low self-esteem related to lack of confidence caused by chronic illness or impairment

DESIRED PATIENT OUTCOME

The child will develop confidence in personal abilities

Outcome measurement criteria

- □ Expression of feelings by the child about the chronic illness and its effects
- □ Expression by the child of a positive self-concept
- □ Participation by the child in family and peer activities
- □ Willingness of the child to assume responsibilities in peer activities
- □ Exhibition by family members and peers of acceptance of the child through hugging, warm interactions, and demonstration of pleasure at being with the child

Key interventions

- Encourage the child and family to express feelings about the child's condition.
- Discuss with the parents ways to increase the child's self-esteem, such as emphasizing and building on the child's strengths; using previously successful activities (if possible) to increase confidence; and praising the child for accomplishments privately and in the presence of siblings and peers.
- Encourage the child's peers to visit, call, and write.
- Teach the child to be honest with peers about the limitations imposed by the chronic condition.
- Enlist the child's teacher and classmates in activities that will enhance the child's self-esteem.
- Help the family and child use support groups or meet people who have similar illnesses or impairments.
- Encourage the parents to actively involve the child in family responsibilities.
- Encourage the family and child to do things together outside the home, if the child's condition permits.
- Realistically discuss with the family the losses that the child and family have suffered because of the chronic condition and the ways in which they can compensate for these losses.

Infant

A child between ages 1 month and 1 year whose physical, psychosocial, and intellectual growth and development are proceeding more rapidly than during any other period after birth.

NURSING DIAGNOSIS

High risk for altered growth and development of the infant

DESIRED PATIENT OUTCOME

The child will demonstrate age-appropriate physical, psychosocial, and intellectual growth and development

Outcome measurement criteria

- ☐ Weight gains of 0.7 to 1 oz (20 to 28 g) per day during the first 6 months and 1 lb (0.45 kg) per month from ages 6 to 12 months; doubling of birth weight by ages 5 to 6 months and tripling of birth weight by age 1 year
- ☐ Length increases of 1" (2.54 cm) per month during the first 6 months and 0.5" (1.27 cm) per month during ages 6 to 12 months; increases of 50% by age 1 year
- ☐ Head circumference increases of 0.5" (1.27 cm) per month during the first 6 months, measuring at least 18.5" (47 cm) by age 1 year
- ☐ Teething beginning at age 6 months and progressing at an average of one tooth per month
- ☐ Motor skill development enabling the infant to turn from the abdomen to the back by age 5 months, sit unsupported by age 8 months, crawl and develop

beginning pincer grasp by age 9 months, creep by age 11 months, and develop refined pincer grasp and walk with assistance by age 12 months

- ☐ Smile at age 2 months in response to social interaction
- ☐ Attachment to primary caregivers and fear of strangers demonstrated by age 8 months
- ☐ Vision demonstrated by eyes following an object or light
- ☐ Hearing demonstrated by head turning toward sound and a startle response
- ☐ Appropriate language skills development, including cooing and babbling by age 3 months, laughing by age 4 months, vocalizing consonant and vowel sounds by age 8 months, and speaking several simple words and understanding many frequently heard words by age 12 months
- ☐ Health and safety needs being met by the parents and caregivers
- ☐ Verbalization by the parents of age-appropriate dietary, sleep, and rest needs
- ☐ Verbalization by the parents of age-appropriate stimulation, exercise, and play activities
- ☐ Development of a sense of trust, according to Erikson's theory
- ☐ Cognitive development appropriate to sensorimotor stage, according to Piaget's theory

Key interventions

- Instruct the parents to supplement breast milk during the first year with fluoride and other minerals or to supplement iron-fortified formula with fluoride, if necessary.
- Advise the parents that infants from ages 1 to 2 months usually drink 21 to 24 oz (621 to 710 ml) of liquid per

day, infants from ages 3 to 6 months drink 30 to 32 oz (887 to 946 ml), and infants who take solid foods drink 24 oz (710 ml).

- Instruct the parents to introduce solid infant foods at ages 4 to 6 months, starting with baby cereal and followed by fruits, vegetables, and meats. Tell them to use a spoon, not a bottle, to feed solid foods; to avoid foods with added salt, sugar, or fat; and to avoid egg white and citrus foods until the infant is age 1 year.
- Advise the parents to encourage drinking from a cup at ages 4 to 6 months and to introduce finger foods, such as crackers, at ages 6 to 7 months.
- Teach the parents to avoid drugs, alcohol, and tobacco and to consult with the primary care practitioner before using medicine when breast-feeding.
- Teach the parents to prepare formula and bottles using clean technique; to hold the bottle when feeding instead of propping it, which could result in choking; and never to leave the infant in bed with a bottle because doing so may lead to tooth decay, ear infections, and choking.
- Teach the parents to provide the infant with adequate opportunities for rest. Explain that a regular bedtime and bedtime ritual are needed, that the infant should sleep in his or her own bed, and that the young infant needs four to six naps daily and the older infant, one or two naps.
- Teach the parents age-appropriate stimulation, exercise, and play activities. For example, advise parents to sing to, hold, and make frequent eye contact with the infant from ages 1 to 3 months; to provide soft toys, play activities, and bath-time activities for the infant from ages 4 to 6 months; to play patty-cake with, provide teething toys for, and talk and laugh with the infant from ages 7 to 9 months; and to provide cloth books, activity toys, and building activities for the infant from ages 10 to 12 months.

- Teach the parents the appropriate infant immunization schedule: diphtheria, tetanus, and pertussis vaccine at ages 2, 4, and 6 months; oral poliovirus vaccine at ages 2 and 4 months; hepatitis B vaccine at birth and ages 1 to 2 months and 6 to 18 months; and *Haemophilus* b conjugate vaccine at ages 2, 4, and 6 months.
- Teach the parents to schedule well-baby checkups at ages 2, 4, 6, and 12 months.
- Teach the parents to provide a safe environment by holding onto the infant when on an elevated surface, such as a changing table or bed; removing dangerous objects from the infant's reach; barricading dangerous areas, such as stairs and hot stoves; ensuring that the crib mattress fits snugly so that the infant will not become wedged between the mattress and crib; inspecting the crib for slats that are too widely spaced; never leaving the infant unattended near pets or in or near water, including toilets and cleaning pails; putting plug covers on electrical outlets; avoiding large crowds when the infant is very young or when contagious diseases are prevalent; and avoiding smoking areas.
- Teach the parents to dress the infant in flame-retardant sleepwear and to lock matches and flammables in a cabinet.
- Teach the parents to use an approved car seat and seat belt for automobile trips and never to leave the infant in a car unattended or during hot weather.

Toddler or preschooler

A child between ages 1 and 2 (toddler) or ages 3 and 5 (preschooler) who is developing physically, psychosocially, and intellectually at a steady but less rapid rate than during infancy.

NURSING DIAGNOSIS

High risk for altered growth and development of the toddler or preschooler

DESIRED PATIENT OUTCOME

The child will demonstrate age-appropriate physical, psychosocial, and intellectual growth and development

Outcome measurement criteria

- ☐ Steady weight gain of approximately 4 to 5 lb (1.8 to 2.3 kg) per year, with quadrupling of birth weight by age 2½
- ☐ Steady height increase of approximately 3" (7.6 cm) per year; height at age 2, when doubled, will approximate adult height
- ☐ Age-appropriate nutrition and feeding, with complete primary dentition (20 teeth) by age 2½ and the ability to use a drinking cup, straw, and spoon at age 2; a fork at age 4; and a table knife for soft foods at age 5
- ☐ Age-appropriate motor skills in the arms, with the ability to build a tower of six blocks by age 2, eight blocks by age 2½, and nine or ten blocks by age 3; to use blunt scissors and copy circles and crosses by age 4; and to catch a ball by age 5

- ☐ Age-appropriate motor skills in the legs, with the ability to walk well without support by age 15 months; run well by ages 24 to 27 months; climb stairs by age 2; jump with both feet by age 2½; ride a tricycle by age 3; jump rope by age 5; and ride a bicycle with training wheels by age 5
- ☐ Age-appropriate toilet training, with daytime bowel and bladder control by age 2½ and the ability to remain dry at night (with only occasional bed-wetting) by age 4
- ☐ Visual acuity of 20/40 by age 4
- ☐ Ability to dress and wash self by age 5
- ☐ Age-appropriate language and conceptual skills, with the ability to use 300 words—including own name, pronouns, familiar items, and body parts—by age 2; understand many regularly heard words, far in excess of speaking vocabulary, throughout the toddler and preschool years; draw a three-part person by age 4; use complete sentences with all parts of speech by age 5; identify at least four colors by age 5; and count to 10 by age 5
- ☐ Age-appropriate play activity, including parallel play at age 2 and associative play at age 3
- ☐ Expression of affection in the form of hugs and kisses throughout the toddler and preschool years
- ☐ Development of a sense of autonomy by a toddler and development of a sense of initiative by a preschooler, according to Erikson's theory
- ☐ Cognitive development appropriate to preoperational stage, according to Piaget's theory
- ☐ Ability to easily separate from parents by age 5
- ☐ Meeting of the infant's health and safety needs by the parents
- ☐ Verbalization by the parents of age-appropriate dietary, sleep, and rest needs

☐ Verbalization by the parents of age-appropriate stimulation, exercise, and play activities

Key interventions

- Advise the parents to begin toilet training after the child can walk well, communicate needs, demonstrate displeasure with wet or dirty diaper, and use fine motor skills to assist in removing clothes. Instruct the parents to begin toilet training during warm weather, when the child will be wearing minimal clothing.
- Teach the parents to initiate bowel training first, using a potty chair or a commode with an attached child's seat and a footstool under the child's feet; to establish a set time each day for the child to sit on the potty chair; and to applaud the child's efforts, whether or not they are successful.
- Teach the parents to initiate daytime bladder training after bowel training by taking the child to the potty chair at regular intervals during the day, telling the child to use the potty when the urge to urinate is present, and praising efforts whether or not they are successful.
- Instruct the parents to initiate nighttime bladder training when the child remains dry all day and expresses displeasure at having to wear a diaper at night.
- Encourage the parents to floss the child's teeth daily and to teach the child how to brush the teeth.
- Teach the parents the appropriate immunization and test schedule for the toddler or preschooler: measles, mumps, and rubella vaccine at age 15 months; tuberculin skin testing at ages 15 months and 4 to 6 years; diphtheria, tetanus, and pertussis vaccine at ages 15 to 18 months and before school entry (ages 4 to 6); oral poliovirus vaccine at ages 15 to 18 months and before school entry (ages 4 to 6); *Haemophilus* b conjugate vaccine at ages 12 to 15 months; and influenza virus vaccine annually for children age 6 months or older who

have a chronic illness, such as asthma or diabetes mellitus.

- Teach the parents to schedule well-child checkups at ages 15 months (or earlier) and 4 years.
- Encourage the parents to schedule annual dental checkups beginning when the child has a full set of primary teeth.
- Teach the parents to feed their toddler or preschooler appropriately. Advise them to include the child in mealtime conversation; provide small servings of vegetables, fruits, meat, and starches (including bread) and then give additional food if desired; provide at least 16 oz (473 ml) of milk daily; provide healthful snacks and allow the child to choose between two healthy options; encourage the child to drink water and juice when thirsty between meals; and include sweets as part of meals, not as between-meal snacks.
- Teach the parents to provide adequate rest opportunities for the child. Encourage them to establish a bedtime ritual and provide a security object, such as a teddy bear or blanket.
- Advise the parents that the child should be allowed to choose between two equally desirable books to read at bedtime, should sleep in the child's own bed, should regularly sleep for 12 hours a night, and may need one or two daily naps if a toddler or one short daily nap if a preschooler.
- Teach the parents to consistently enforce rules, use the time-out method (in which the misbehaving child must sit apart or abstain from play) for 1 minute for each year of age, and provide opportunities for the child to make healthy choices, such as choosing which of two vegetables to eat.
- Teach the parents to provide a safe environment by checking bathwater temperature and not allowing the child to draw bathwater or turn on faucets; barricading

dangerous areas; removing sharp items, firearms and ammunition, plastic bags, and other harmful objects from the child's reach; placing plug covers on electrical outlets; avoiding large crowds when contagious diseases are prevalent; avoiding smoking areas; and fencing and locking any home swimming area.

- Teach the parents to dress the child in flame-retardant sleepwear and lock away matches and other flammables.
- Teach the parents to involve the child in safety measures by teaching the child the full name and address, instructing the child to avoid strangers, requiring the child to wear a seat belt when in an automobile or bus, insisting on safe street crossing behaviors, requiring that the child play in a fenced yard, and teaching swimming and water safety at age 6 or earlier.
- Teach the parents appropriate exercise, play, and social activities for the toddler or preschooler. Recommend fill-and-empty and push-pull toys, such as a wagon or shopping cart; large balls; cardboard boxes; puzzles and other problem-solving toys; picture books; stuffed animals with secure eyes, noses, and other ornamentation; a child's set of pots and pans and replicas of other adult household objects, such as tools and clothing; coloring and drawing materials; and a tricycle and helmet.
- Advise the parents to include the child in family activities, such as mealtime conversation and family discussions.
- Recommend that the parents limit television viewing to brief sessions of children's educational programs.
- Advise the parents to talk, laugh, and read with the child; to encourage music and singing; and to provide opportunities for play with other children.
- Encourage the parents to praise the child for participation in positive play activities.

School-age child

A child between ages 6 and 12 who is developing physically, psychosocially, and intellectually at a faster rate than during the toddler and preschooler years.

NURSING DIAGNOSIS

High risk for altered growth and development of the school-age child

DESIRED PATIENT OUTCOME

The child will demonstrate age-appropriate physical, psychosocial, and intellectual growth and development

Outcome measurement criteria

- ☐ Ability to dress self appropriately
- ☐ Performance of personal hygiene
- ☐ Consumption of nutritious meals and healthful snacks
- ☐ Absence of major injuries because of carelessness or accidents
- ☐ Maintenance of physical health with no major illnesses
- ☐ Maintenance of dental health with no dental caries
- ☐ Development of a sense of industry, according to Erikson's theory
- ☐ Cognitive development in the area of concrete operations, according to Piaget's theory
- ☐ Maintenance of passing school grades
- ☐ Acceptance of a responsible family role as exhibited by performance of assigned tasks

Key interventions

- Encourage the parents to guide clothing choices until the child learns to dress appropriately.
- Teach the child body, hair, and dental hygiene, instructing the child to wash the body (including the neck, ears, face, and underarms) daily and thoroughly with soap, to wash hair every other day with shampoo and rinse thoroughly, and to brush teeth and floss morning and night.
- Teach the child to eat appropriate foods from the food pyramid for meals and snacks.
- Encourage the child to assist with meal preparation and to enjoy family interaction at mealtime.
- Emphasize skateboard, bicycle, motor bike, and automobile safety, such as wearing a helmet or seat belt.
- Teach water safety rules, such as checking the water's depth before diving, always swimming with a partner, and avoiding horseplay.
- Teach precautions to take with strangers, such as keeping doors locked; refusing to open the door when home alone unless the visitor is a close family member; never telling a telephone caller that the child is alone; refusing to talk to or get near strangers under any circumstances; and letting parents or teachers know if an older child or adult says or does things that are disturbing, such as touching private body areas.
- Teach the parents to have their child immunized against measles, mumps, and rubella at ages 11 to 12.
- Teach the parents to provide for adequate rest. Explain that the child needs 10 to 11 hours of sleep at night and that a regular bedtime and bedtime ritual (such as bathing and going to bed by 8:30 p.m.) should be established.

- Teach the parents appropriate exercise, play, and social activities for their child. Advise them to encourage fair play and reward activities that exhibit honesty and respect for others; encourage the use of toys and activities that develop fine motor skills and a sense of accomplishment and success, such as building blocks, puzzles, models, puppets, and art projects; encourage play that develops large motor skills, social skills, and relationship skills, such as team sports, jumping rope, hide-and-seek, hiking, and playing with a pet; limit television viewing to brief periods and appropriate programs; and provide opportunities for social activities with friends, such as spending the night with a friend or attending a birthday party.
- Teach the dangers of high-risk behavior, such as smoking, taking drugs, drinking alcohol, playing with or using guns, and engaging in sexual activities. Keep communication pathways open with the child, encouraging questions and information sharing.
- Encourage the parents to teach good study habits and provide opportunities for cognitive and creative activities. Advise them to discuss the child's interests and assist the child in pursuing them; to provide a quiet area for homework; to encourage the child to plan, so that projects, homework, and studies are completed in advance; to provide opportunities for the child to demonstrate reading, writing, and mathematical skills; to reward cognitive and creative accomplishments by providing praise and displaying artwork, report cards, and other efforts; and to take the child to museums and cultural events and then discuss what was seen.
- Encourage the parents to assign the child regular household tasks and to provide positive reinforcement, such as praise or a small allowance, for completion of tasks.

Adolescent

An individual between ages 13 and 18 who is developing physically, psychosocially, and intellectually at a rapid rate.

NURSING DIAGNOSIS

High risk for altered growth and development of the adolescent

DESIRED PATIENT OUTCOME

The child will demonstrate age-appropriate physical, psychosocial, and intellectual growth and development

Outcome measurement criteria

- ☐ Responsible management of self-care, such as eating nutritious foods, dressing appropriately, sleeping enough, maintaining proper physical and dental hygiene, and exercising adequately
- ☐ Absence of alcohol, drug, or tobacco use
- ☐ Absence of major injuries because of accidents
- ☐ Maintenance of physical health with no serious illnesses
- ☐ Maintenance of dental health with no dental caries
- ☐ Maintenance of passing grades in school
- ☐ Development of a sense of identity, according to Erikson's theory
- ☐ Ability to perform abstract operations, according to Piaget's theory

Key interventions

- Teach the parents the importance of the adolescent's assuming responsibility for personal nutrition, rest, hygiene, and exercise.

- Encourage the parents to schedule regular medical and dental checkups for the adolescent.
- Teach cancer screening techniques, including breast self-examination for girls and testicular self-examination for boys.
- Provide scoliosis screening at ages 14 and 16.
- Teach the parents the importance of immunizing the adolescent against tetanus and diphtheria at ages 14 to 16 and against hepatitis unless a vaccine was given earlier in childhood.
- Teach the parents the importance of having the adolescent tested for tuberculosis at age 15 or 16.
- Provide information about skin care to reduce acne.
- Provide information about alcohol and drug abuse.
- Provide information about sex and sexually transmitted diseases.
- Encourage the parents to provide driver education lessons and positive reinforcement for good driving behaviors.
- Encourage the parents to provide positive reinforcement, such as praise, special treats or gifts, or extra allowance, for good school performance.
- Encourage the parents to provide opportunities for the adolescent to be with peers in safe, healthy situations, such as chaperoned parties, church or club activities, and school events.
- Advise the parents to encourage the adolescent's special interests and provide recognition for activities participation, awards, and honors.
- Advise the parents to include the adolescent in family discussions and problem solving by assigning regular chores, recognizing and rewarding responsible behavior, encouraging limited outside employment and organizational activities, and providing an allowance to develop money management abilities.

Diabetes mellitus, insulin-dependent

A metabolic disorder in which a lack of insulin prevents carbohydrates from being appropriately metabolized, causing such initial symptoms as polydipsia, polyuria, and polyphagia.

NURSING DIAGNOSIS

Anxiety related to lack of knowledge about diabetes mellitus

DESIRED PATIENT OUTCOME

The parents and child will demonstrate increased knowledge and reduced anxiety about the child's disease and care

Outcome measurement criteria

- ☐ Verbalization by the parents of increased comfort with the child's condition
- ☐ Return to normal sleeping patterns by all family members
- ☐ Resumption by all family members of appropriate developmental tasks
- ☐ Verbalization by the parents of the role of insulin in glucose metabolism
- ☐ Verbalization by the parents (and child, if age-appropriate) of the major signs and symptoms of diabetes mellitus
- ☐ Verbalization by the parents of how the child's diabetes mellitus will affect the family unit and each family member

Key interventions

- Assess the child's and family's previous experiences with hospitalization.
- Orient the child and parents to the hospital and its routine.
- Teach the parents to encourage the child and any siblings to deal with anxiety by using play.
- Encourage open communication among family members and between the nurse and family members. Urge them to express their fears and concerns.
- Assess the return to the usual family routines and patterns, such as sleeping, eating, and working.
- Encourage the parents to spend as much time as possible with the child.
- Explain to the parents and child (if age-appropriate) the purpose of laboratory tests.
- Provide the parents and child (if age-appropriate) with general information about the child's condition, gradually adding specific information to prepare them for the child's discharge.
- Discuss with the parents the necessary changes in the family's and child's lifestyles, including how diet, medications, exercise, medical expenses, glucose testing, and caregiver responsibilities will affect the child and family.

NURSING DIAGNOSIS

Altered nutrition: less than body requirements, related to lack of knowledge about diet for diabetes mellitus

DESIRED PATIENT OUTCOME

The parents and child will adhere to appropriate dietary management principles

Outcome measurement criteria

- ☐ Verbalization by the parents of the relation between diet and disease management
- ☐ Maintenance of the blood glucose level between 80 and 120 mg/dl
- ☐ Verbalization by the parents of an understanding of the food pyramid and the basics of the child's dietary plan
- ☐ Development by the parents of a sample diet, including snacks, that reflects the child's caloric requirements
- ☐ Verbalization by the child (if age-appropriate) that the new diet is acceptable
- ☐ Weight appropriate for the child's age

Key interventions

- Teach the parents and the child about the relation of diet, insulin, and glucose levels.
- Refer the family and child to a dietitian for initial dietary instructions.
- Follow up on dietary instructions, reviewing sample diets for appropriate calories and use of the food pyramid.
- Check that the child's diet includes cultural food preferences as much as possible.
- Ask the parents and child (if age-appropriate) about the child's food preferences, and suggest sugar-free versions of favorite foods, if available.
- Teach the parents to eliminate, as much as possible, concentrated sweets from the child's diet and to limit dietary fat intake to no more than 30%.
- Tell the parents to provide the child with extra snacks, such as cheese or peanut butter with crackers, if additional physical exercise is planned.

- Encourage the child (if age-appropriate) to assist in planning meals and snacks; discuss the acceptability of the diet with the child.
- Monitor the child's weight and blood glucose level.

NURSING DIAGNOSIS

High risk for injury related to insufficient glucose (hypoglycemia) or excessive glucose (hyperglycemia)

DESIRED PATIENT OUTCOME

The child will not experience hypoglycemia or hyperglycemia

Outcome measurement criteria

- ☐ Verbalization by the parents of the causes of hypoglycemia and hyperglycemia
- ☐ Identification by the parents and child (if age-appropriate) of the signs and symptoms of hypoglycemia and hyperglycemia
- ☐ Verbalization by the parents and child (if age-appropriate) of the treatments for hypoglycemia and hyperglycemia
- ☐ Maintenance of blood glucose level between 80 and 120 mg/dl
- ☐ Urine negative for ketones
- ☐ Absence of injury to the child as a result of therapy
- ☐ Wearing by the child of a medical identification necklace or bracelet

Key interventions

- Inform the parents that hypoglycemia results from one or more of the following: excessive exercise, too little food, illness, too much insulin.

- Teach the parents and child (if age-appropriate) the signs and symptoms of hypoglycemia, such as rapid pulse, hunger, shakiness, dizziness, anxiety, irritability, pallor, moist skin, poor concentration, and confusion.
- Teach the parents and child (if age-appropriate) that hypoglycemia should be treated, if the child is conscious, by feeding the child sugar candies, table sugar, sugar cubes, honey, or soft drinks or juices containing sugar.
- Explain to the parents and child (if age-appropriate) that if hypoglycemia is not relieved within 15 minutes, the child should again eat sugar-laden foods, followed by cheese and crackers or a peanut butter sandwich.
- Teach the parents to give glucagon by injection if the child is unconscious or unable to swallow and notify the primary care practitioner.
- Inform the parents that hyperglycemia results from improper diet, inadequate insulin, illness, or a combination of these factors.
- Teach the parents and child (if age-appropriate) to recognize the signs and symptoms of hyperglycemia, including lethargy, confusion, unconsciousness, thirst, flushed skin, fruity-smelling breath, excessive urination, dehydration, abdominal pain, and vomiting.
- Teach the parents and child (if age-appropriate) how to give insulin injections. Demonstrate sterile technique, explain how to accurately measure and mix insulin, instruct on rotating injection sites, and have the parents and child practice the injection technique on a cloth doll or orange.
- Instruct the parents and child (if age-appropriate) to check the blood glucose level before meals and at bedtime. Explain the blood glucose test to the child in a developmentally appropriate manner.

- Always wear gloves when conducting the blood glucose test, and teach the parents to wear gloves when conducting the test if the child is positive for human immunodeficiency virus or hepatitis B virus.
- Tell the parents and child (if age-appropriate) to check the expiration date on the bottle containing the blood glucose test strips and not to use them if the date has passed.
- Advise the parents and child (if age-appropriate) that the proper test site is on the side of the heel for infants and on the side of the fingertip or earlobe for children.
- Teach the parents and child (if age-appropriate) how to administer the blood glucose test. Instruct them to clean the test site with alcohol, allow the alcohol to dry, and then prick the site. Advise them to wipe away the first drop of blood using dry gauze, to place the second drop of blood on the reagent pad, and then to apply pressure on the prick site. Tell them to follow bottle directions for the timing and color code if using glucose test strips and to follow directions for operation if using a blood glucose meter (Glucometer).
- Instruct the parents to notify the primary care practitioner if the blood glucose level is below 40 or above 240 mg/dl.
- Advise the parents to check the child's urine for ketones if the blood glucose level is above 240 mg/dl or if the child is ill.
- Tell the parents and child (if age-appropriate) to record glucose and ketone readings, insulin doses, injection sites, diet, and any illness.
- Explain to the parents that stress and illness may increase the child's insulin needs and that exercise will reduce insulin needs.
- Teach the parents and child (if age-appropriate) about the effects of uncontrolled diabetes.

- Request that the parents require the child to wear a medical identification bracelet or necklace.

NURSING DIAGNOSIS

High risk for caregiver role strain related to the stress of caring for a child with diabetes mellitus

DESIRED PATIENT OUTCOME

The parents and child (if age-appropriate) will successfully implement home care

Outcome measurement criteria

- ☐ Verbalization by the parents of the information they will need for successful home care
- ☐ Verbalization by the parents of the problems they will encounter in caring for the child at home and ways to manage these problems
- ☐ Expression by the parents of feelings about home care
- ☐ Verbalization by the parents and child (if age-appropriate) of satisfaction with the home-care situation
- ☐ Use by the parents of recommended community and family resources
- ☐ Absence of child hospitalization caused by inadequate home care

Key interventions

- Refer the family to a dietitian, who will explain initial dietary management principles.
- Review diet plans with the family.
- Teach the parents and child (if age-appropriate) the signs and symptoms of abnormally low and abnormally high glucose and how to intervene when glucose is low or high.

- Advise the parents and child (if age-appropriate) about the importance of prompt care for injuries and infections and good oral and skin hygiene.
- Teach the parents and child (if age-appropriate) how to give insulin injections and how to adjust food and insulin intake to exercise patterns.
- Teach the parents and child (if age-appropriate) how to test for urine ketones and blood glucose.
- Provide the parents with written materials to take home that discuss the points taught during the child's hospitalization.
- Discuss the problems of home care, such as caregiving if both parents work; the costs of insulin, glucose and urine monitoring, and medical visits; and arranging for transportation to and attendance at follow-up visits.
- Develop a plan to provide the child's home care, involving all immediate family members and any available extended family members.
- Support and encourage the family members and child as they learn the aspects of care.
- Provide the phone number of the health care facility so that the family can call the nurse with questions about treatment.
- Inform the family about available community resources.
- Encourage the parents to express feelings about home care.

NURSING DIAGNOSIS

Altered growth and development related to the effects of hospitalization and treatment of diabetes mellitus

DESIRED PATIENT OUTCOME

The child will display normal physical and mental development

Outcome measurement criteria

- ☐ Verbalization by the parents of age-appropriate growth and development norms for the child
- ☐ Verbalization by the parents of the effects of diabetes mellitus on normal growth and development
- ☐ Age-appropriate growth and development of the child, including social, communication, and intellectual skills

Key interventions

- Teach the parents growth and development norms for the child.
- Instruct the parents about the key aspects of managing the child's disease, including diet, exercise, and insulin administration.
- Teach the parents the relation between managing the child's diabetes mellitus and growth and development.
- Inform the parents that lack of adherence to the therapeutic regimen results in hospitalization, injury, or both and that hospitalization reduces the child's participation in school and daily activities.
- Tell the parents to manage the disease by setting limits for the child. Advise them to use positive reinforcement methods.
- Assess the child's growth pattern at regular intervals.
- Assess the child's social, communication, and intellectual skills annually.

Hypothyroidism, congenital

A thyroid hormone deficiency that is present at birth and affects a child's growth and development.

NURSING DIAGNOSIS

Anxiety related to insufficient parental knowledge about congenital hypothyroidism (CH)

DESIRED PATIENT OUTCOME

The parents will demonstrate increased knowledge of and reduced anxiety about CH

Outcome measurement criteria

- ☐ Verbalization by the parents of knowledge about CH
- ☐ Description by the parents of the early signs of CH
- ☐ Prompt reporting by the parents of signs of thyroid deficiency
- ☐ Genetic counseling obtained by the parents if the child displays signs of CH

Key interventions

- Encourage the parents to express fears and concerns about their child's condition.
- Be aware that infants who were not born in a health care facility may not have received the CH screening test.
- Inform the parents that even though CH screening is performed shortly after birth in most states, they should be alert to signs of CH.

- Tell the parents that signs of CH appear at approximately age 6 weeks in bottle-fed babies and after weaning in breast-fed babies and include a short forehead and hirsutism; coarse, dry, and dull hair; a short nose with a depressed nasal bridge; a puffy face and eyelids; jaundice during the first weeks of life; dry, cool, thickened skin; mottled appearance; a large, protruding tongue; a large, protruding abdomen; constipation; poor eating; very little crying; chronic sleepiness or excessive sleeping; and fatigue and inactivity.
- Advise the parents to inform the primary care practitioner if the child exhibits signs of CH.
- Explain to the parents that certain types of hypothyroidism may be inherited and that parents of affected infants should seek genetic counseling.

NURSING DIAGNOSIS

Altered health maintenance related to lack of parental knowledge about care of the child with CH

DESIRED PATIENT OUTCOME

The parents will provide appropriate care for the child with CH

Outcome measurement criteria

- ☐ Verbalization by the parents of why the child needs thyroid medication
- ☐ Identification of medication considerations
- ☐ Demonstration of proper pulse measurement
- ☐ Absence in the child of signs and symptoms of thyroid medication overdose
- ☐ Consistent maintaining by the parents of follow-up appointments for the child
- ☐ Age-appropriate growth and development of the child

□ Alertness and participation by the child in play

Key interventions

- Explain that the child must take thyroid medication for life and that mental retardation will occur without it.
- Explain that the child's need for thyroid hormone may increase during growth spurts and other periods and that the dosage may have to be adjusted.
- Teach the parents to take the child's pulse.
- Discuss how to give oral thyroid medication by crushing medication in tablet form, giving medication early in the morning and when the child's stomach is empty, and checking the child's pulse before giving medication. Advise the parents to withhold medication and report an abnormally high pulse rate.
- Explain that signs of hypothyroidism will disappear after months of taking thyroid medication and that any mental damage can be arrested but not repaired.
- Advise the parents to call the primary care practitioner if the child develops signs of thyroid overdose, such as restlessness, sleeplessness, and weight loss.
- Teach the parents the age-appropriate diet for the child.
- Warn the parents to feed the child slowly, with the head elevated, to prevent choking on formula or food. Teach the abdominal thrust (Heimlich maneuver).
- Instruct the parents to prevent constipation by giving extra fluids and a stool softener, if prescribed.
- Urge the parents to return the child regularly for blood tests and growth and development monitoring.
- Teach the parents appropriate stimulation, exercise, and play activities for the child.

Phenylketonuria

An inherited absence of phenylalanine hydroxylase, an amino acid necessary for breakdown of the amino acid tyrosine, which causes a high serum level of phenylalanine and the presence of phenyl acids in the urine. Without treatment, mental retardation results.

NURSING DIAGNOSIS

Anticipatory grieving (parental) related to the potential loss of the child's health because of phenylketonuria (PKU)

DESIRED PATIENT OUTCOME

The parents will appropriately resolve the grief associated with the potential loss of the child's health

Outcome measurement criteria

- ☐ Verbalization by the parents that reflects an understanding of the stages of grief
- ☐ Expression of grief by the parents
- ☐ Verbalization by the parents of how caring for the child will alter the life-style of the family as a unit and as individuals
- ☐ Verbalization by the parents of a plan to manage the initial phases of the child's PKU
- ☐ Demonstration by the family members of mutual support, such as holding one another and talking openly about feelings

Key interventions

- Assess the family's past experiences with grief and loss and determine if the grief was successfully resolved.

- Explain that grieving is normal, and clarify any misconceptions about grief.
- Identify the strengths of the family as a unit and as individuals.
- Encourage family members to discuss their feelings about the diagnosis of PKU and loss of the child's health.
- Encourage the parents to be open and truthful with all family members, including the child.
- Prepare the parents for possible responses of people outside the immediate family on hearing the diagnosis of PKU.
- Discuss ways to manage the immediate details of caring for a chronically ill child, including care of other children in the family, arrangements with employers, financial considerations, and necessary modifications to the home environment.
- Involve the family in a support group.
- Encourage the family to demonstrate love and support of one another.

NURSING DIAGNOSIS

Altered growth and development related to insufficient parental knowledge about PKU

DESIRED PATIENT OUTCOME

The child will experience normal physical and mental development

Outcome measurement criteria

☐ Verbalization by the parents of knowledge of the effects of untreated PKU on the child's mental development

☐ Description by the parents of the early signs and symptoms of PKU

☐ Prompt attention by the parents to signs and symptoms of PKU by taking the child to a primary care practitioner

Key interventions

- Be aware that children who were not born in a health care facility may not have received a PKU screening test.
- Teach the parents that, if untreated, PKU will arrest the child's mental development.
- Teach the patients to recognize and report signs and symptoms of PKU, such as musty body odor, frequent vomiting, erratic behavior, and irritability.
- Check the child for normal growth and development. If development is delayed, question the parents about specific PKU signs and symptoms, and check the child's record for PKU screening results.

NURSING DIAGNOSIS

Altered health maintenance related to lack of knowledge about care of the child with PKU

DESIRED PATIENT OUTCOME

The parents will provide age-appropriate care for the child with PKU

Outcome measurement criteria

☐ Verbalization by the parents of knowledge about PKU, including its hereditary origin

☐ Genetic counseling obtained by the parents

☐ Genetic counseling obtained for the child, if an adolescent

☐ Verbalization by the parents of the need for a special diet for the child with PKU

- ☐ Development by the parents of a menu low in phenylalanine
- ☐ Consistent maintenance by the parents of follow-up appointments for the child
- ☐ Age-appropriate growth and development of the child

Key interventions

- Explain to the parents and child (if age-appropriate) about PKU and the role of heredity in the disease.
- Encourage the parents to seek genetic counseling for themselves and the child, if an adolescent.
- Instruct the parents and child (if age-appropriate) about the need for a low-phenylalanine diet. Explain that such a diet must be continued through adolescence and must be resumed by women before pregnancy.
- Refer the parents to a dietitian for consultation, and reinforce dietary instructions.
- Teach that breast-feeding is acceptable because breast milk is low in phenylalanine.
- Inform the parents that low-phenylalanine formulas (such as Lofenalac) are available for infants and that phenylalanine-free formulas (such as Phenyl-free and PKU2) are available for children over age 1. Explain that phenylalanine-free formulas allow more food intake because they contain no phenylalanine and that low-phenylalanine and phenylalanine-free formulas have a strong taste and odor and are expensive.
- Teach that solid foods containing large quantities of phenylalanine, such as meat, green vegetables, eggs, and dairy products, should be avoided.
- Explain that foods containing aspartame (Nutrasweet) should be avoided because the body converts aspartame to phenylalanine.

- Explain that the intake of low-phenylalanine foods, such as fruits, some vegetables, and breads and other starches, must be carefully monitored so that an acceptable serum phenylalanine level is obtained. Also explain that high-calorie foods in this group are needed to maintain adequate growth.
- Teach the parents and child (if age-appropriate) about dietary restrictions and how to read food labels.
- Advise the parents to inform the child's teachers about PKU and dietary restrictions.
- Encourage the parents to have the child's condition and growth and development monitored regularly during follow-up visits.

Cleft lip and palate

Congenital defects of the lip and palate caused by nonunion of embryonic facial structures that may occur together or separately.

NURSING DIAGNOSIS

Anticipatory grieving (parental) related to loss of the child's health

DESIRED PATIENT OUTCOME

The parents will cope effectively with the grief associated with loss of the child's health

Outcome measurement criteria

- ☐ Verbalization by the parents of understanding of grief
- ☐ Expressions of grief by the parents
- ☐ Verbalization by the parents of support for each other
- ☐ Verbalization by the extended family of support for the parents
- ☐ Verbalization by the parents that the child's lip or palate can be repaired
- ☐ Identification by the parents of a plan to manage the initial phases of their adjustment to the situation

Key interventions

- Assess the family's past experiences with grief and loss and determine if grief was resolved successfully.
- Explain that grieving is normal, and clarify any misconceptions about grief.

- Encourage the parents to express their feelings about the congenital defect and loss of the child's health.
- Encourage the parents to be open and truthful with other family members.
- Prepare the parents for possible responses to the child's cleft lip or cleft palate by people outside the immediate family.
- Identify the strengths of the family as a unit and as individuals.
- Encourage family members to demonstrate love and support for one another.
- Provide initial information about cleft lip and cleft palate, explaining that these conditions can be repaired. Teach that cleft lip is repaired when the child is between ages 1 and 3 months, that initial cleft palate repair is performed at about age 18 months and before significant speech development occurs, and that, depending on the size of the palate defect, several subsequent repairs may be needed.
- Discuss ways of managing the immediate situation, including caring for the family's other children, making arrangements with employers, and planning for financial considerations.

NURSING DIAGNOSIS

Altered parenting related to impaired parent-infant attachment

DESIRED PATIENT OUTCOME

The parents will develop satisfactory attachment to the infant

Outcome measurement criteria

□ Participation by the parents in the child's care

- ☐ Verbalization by the parents of positive feelings toward the child
- ☐ Demonstration of positive parental interactions, such as frequent eye contact and holding, stroking, and cuddling of the child
- ☐ Verbalization by parents of optimism about the outcome of the child's treatment
- ☐ Use by parents of community support systems
- ☐ Age-appropriate growth and development of the child

Key interventions

- Demonstrate a positive reaction to the child.
- Emphasize the child's positive characteristics, such as beautiful eyes and hands, rather than focusing on the cleft lip or cleft palate.
- Encourage the parents, as well as the extended family and friends, to participate in the child's care as soon as possible.
- Encourage the parents to express their feelings.
- Provide opportunities for the parents to hold and interact with the child.
- Reinforce positive parental interactions, such as eye contact, cuddling, and holding.
- Express optimism about the possibility of successfully repairing the cleft lip or cleft palate.
- Arrange for the parents to visit with the parent of a child who has had a similar condition.
- Refer the family to a support group, clergy member, or both, if the family desires.
- Teach the parents about normal growth and developmental milestones. Assess the child's growth and development at regular follow-up visits.

Nursing Diagnosis

Altered nutrition: less than body requirements, related to impaired feeding ability

DESIRED PATIENT OUTCOME

The child will obtain adequate nutrition

Outcome measurement criteria

- ☐ Weight gain of 1 oz (28 g) per day after the expected 10% initial weight loss shortly after birth
- ☐ Increased parental confidence in feeding the child
- ☐ No instances of choking during feeding or expelling formula through the nose
- ☐ Displays of contentment by the child between feedings

Key interventions

- Assess whether preoperative breast-feeding is possible. If the mother plans to breast-feed, arrange for someone who is experienced in breast-feeding infants with cleft lip or cleft palate, such as a member of La Leche League, to contact the mother.
- Demonstrate to the parents the appropriate preoperative bottle- or large-syringe–feeding technique for an infant with cleft lip or cleft palate. Advise parents to position the child with the head nearly upright; to use a long, soft nipple or tubing attached to a large syringe, whichever is appropriate; to place the nipple or tube on the side opposite the cleft; and to drip milk into the child's mouth slowly, controlling the flow and allowing the child to suck. Explain that milk should be deposited at the back of the child's mouth to reduce the possibility of it entering the nasal cavity. Advise parents using a nipple to remove it only for burping or if the child is choking.

- Explain that infants with cleft lip or cleft palate tend to swallow a great deal of air and that parents should burp the child after every 0.5 oz (14 g) of feeding.
- Teach the parents to rinse milk from the cleft by giving water after each feeding, to limit feeding to 30 minutes, and to position the infant in a semisitting position after feeding.
- Demonstrate any special feeding devices, such as a nipple with a flange that occludes the cleft or a lamb's nipple (a big, soft nipple with large holes), to the parents. Allow them to gain confidence in using the devices before the child's discharge.
- Have both parents demonstrate feeding the child, giving positive reinforcement and assisting if the child begins to choke or cough.
- Keep a fluid intake and output record for the hospitalized child, and teach the parents of the bottle-fed child to record the number of ounces (grams) taken at each feeding.
- Before surgery, teach the child with a cleft palate to drink from a cup or the side of a spoon and to eat small amounts of baby food from a spoon by ages 4 to 6 months. Introduce new foods one at a time every 4 days.
- Weigh the hospitalized child daily at the same time, using the same scale, and while the child is undressed. Instruct the parents to weigh the child weekly on the same day and to keep a record of the weight.
- Teach the parents the appropriate postoperative feeding techniques. Advise the parents of a child who has had a cleft lip repaired to feed the child in an upright position, making frequent eye contact; to use tubing and a large syringe initially for feeding, placing the tubing in the side of the mouth and avoiding the suture line; to feed clear liquids initially, gradually adding formula; to burp the child after every 0.5 oz (14 g); to rinse milk or formula from the cleft by giving water after each feed-

ing; to position the infant in a semisitting position, preferably slanted to the right side, after feeding; and to note whether the child is retaining feedings.

- Teach the parents of the child who has had a cleft palate repaired to feed small amounts of clear liquids initially, then a full liquid diet, and finally a soft diet approximately 3 weeks after surgery; to give fluids initially from a cup, the side of a large spoon, or a tube attached to a large syringe; to document the child's tolerance of food and liquid intake; to rinse the infant's mouth by giving water after each feeding; and not to place any object, such as a bottle, nipple, spoon, fork, or straw, in the child's mouth for the first 3 weeks after surgery.
- Assess the child's behavior immediately after and between feedings. Note the child's degree of contentment and ability to sleep.

NURSING DIAGNOSIS

High risk for injury related to infection

DESIRED PATIENT OUTCOME

The child will display no signs or symptoms of infection

Outcome measurement criteria

- ☐ Light pink or gray tympanic membranes
- ☐ Clear lung sounds
- ☐ Temperature below 100° F (37.8° C)
- ☐ Pink, intact skin and mucous membrane at cleft site preoperatively
- ☐ Pink, approximated suture line of lip, palate, or both postoperatively

Key interventions

- Emphasize to the parents that using the appropriate feeding technique helps prevent aspiration and ear infections.
- Place the child in a semisitting position and on the right side after feeding.
- Examine the tympanic membranes for signs of infection before discharge and at each follow-up visit.
- Auscultate the hospitalized child's lung fields every 4 hours.
- Check the child's temperature every 4 hours during hospitalization and when indicated after discharge.
- Rinse the child's mouth by giving water after each feeding.
- Remove dried milk from the cleft by using a moistened applicator. While doing this, assess the mucous membranes and skin.
- Carefully clean the lip suture line with a solution as ordered; apply antibiotic ointment, if prescribed.

NURSING DIAGNOSIS

High risk for injury (to operative repair sites) related to the child's mobility and the parents' lack of knowledge about postoperative care

DESIRED PATIENT OUTCOME

The child will heal appropriately at operative repair sites

Outcome measurement criteria

- ☐ Lip suture line that remains approximated as it heals
- ☐ Barely noticeable lip scar
- ☐ Cleft palate suture line that remains approximated as it heals

Key interventions

- Confirm that the Logan bow or butterfly tape dressing is in place after cleft lip surgery.
- Place the child on the side after cleft lip surgery.
- Consult with the parents before cleft lip surgery to determine the usual consoling techniques; use these techniques to soothe the child after surgery to prevent excessive crying or stressing of the suture line.
- Use elbow restraints to prevent the child's hands from touching the repaired cleft lip; release the restraints one at a time every 2 hours and exercise the arms.
- Use a jacket restraint to prevent the child who has had cleft lip surgery from turning onto the abdomen. If possible and safe, apply the jacket restraint so that the child can be placed in a side-lying position to facilitate postsurgical drainage and positioning after feeding. Remove the restraint for 15 minutes every 2 hours and then replace it. (Be sure to supervise the child when the restraint is removed.)
- Encourage the parents of a child using a jacket restraint to hold the child when he or she is not wearing the restraint. Advise them that the restraint must be in place whenever they are not holding the child.
- Carefully monitor the child wearing a jacket restraint to prevent injury.
- Clean the lip suture line using a solution as ordered; apply ointment if prescribed.
- Assess the lip suture line for signs of infection and for approximation.
- Place the child who has had cleft palate surgery in a mist tent during the immediate postoperative period, turning the child every 2 hours.
- Facilitate drainage flow by placing the child who has had cleft palate surgery on the abdomen or side.

- Use elbow restraints to prevent the child who has had cleft palate surgery from putting fingers or objects into the mouth; release the restraints one at a time every 2 hours to exercise the arms.
- Observe the respiratory status of the child who has had cleft palate surgery every 15 minutes initially, then every hour, and then every 4 hours. Auscultate the lung fields, and be alert for signs of distress, such as cyanosis, retractions, and flaring of nares.
- Take vital signs every 15 minutes immediately after cleft palate surgery, then every hour, and then every 4 hours.
- Do not suction inside the mouth of the child who has had cleft palate surgery unless an emergency situation, such as an obstructed airway, exists. Do not use a tongue blade in the child's mouth.

NURSING DIAGNOSIS

High risk for caregiver role strain related to long-term home care

DESIRED PATIENT OUTCOME

The parents will manage home care successfully

Outcome measurement criteria

- ☐ Verbalization by the parents of the problems they will encounter in caring for the child at home
- ☐ Identification by the parents of information they will need for successful home care
- ☐ Verbalization by the parents of satisfaction with the home care situation
- ☐ Absence of illness or hospitalization of the child because of inadequate care at home
- ☐ Use by the parents of recommended community and health care resources

- ☐ Weight gain by the child that is consistent with growth norms
- ☐ Accomplishment of age-appropriate developmental tasks by the child

Key interventions

- Encourage the parents to participate in the child's care as much as possible, and assist the parents in learning care techniques.
- Teach the parents the appropriate preoperative and postoperative feeding methods, ways to prevent cleft and middle ear infections, how to protect suture lines during the 4- to 6-week postoperative healing period, the need for follow-up care with the health care team, the possibility of additional surgery, the need for routine immunizations, and the long-term need for frequent dental care, speech therapy, and regular hearing assessment.
- Refer the family to agencies that can assist them, such as the American Cleft Palate Association, the March of Dimes, and state programs that assist the families of children with special needs.
- Assess the child's weight, other indications of growth, and achievement of developmental milestones at scheduled follow-up visits.

Communication or sensory impairment

Difficulty in sending and receiving verbal messages.

NURSING DIAGNOSIS

Impaired verbal communication related to articulation problems, sensory problems, or both

DESIRED PATIENT OUTCOME

The child will demonstrate an improved ability to send or receive messages, or both

Outcome measurement criteria

- ☐ Demonstration of an improved speech pattern
- ☐ Indication of an understanding of verbal communication
- ☐ Appropriate responses to messages sent by others
- ☐ Use of appropriate assistive techniques or devices, such as an electronic larynx, a hearing aid, sign language, and Braille script, if needed
- ☐ Use by the family of appropriate community support agencies

Key interventions

- Encourage the parents to use an identifying sign, such as a touch, hand squeeze, or kiss, to establish communication with the child.
- Advise the parents to hold the child closely so that the child can feel their speech vibrations.

- Suggest that the parent place the child's hands on the parent's face as a means for the child to communicate.
- Have a specialist evaluate the child to determine whether assistive devices, such as an electronic larynx for the preschool-age or older child, will be helpful.
- Recommend the child for special therapy, such as speech therapy or Braille or sign language instruction.
- Enroll the child in an early intervention program, and contact the local school system about programs available to assist the child and family.

Myringotomy

Incision in the tympanic membrane, usually followed by insertion of drainage tubes.

NURSING DIAGNOSIS

Anxiety related to lack of knowledge about myringotomy and follow-up care

DESIRED PATIENT OUTCOME

The parents will demonstrate increased knowledge and reduced anxiety about the child's surgery and follow-up care

Outcome measurement criteria

- ☐ Verbalization by the parents of the basic aspects of the surgical procedure and the preoperative routine
- ☐ Participation by the parents in immediate postoperative care
- ☐ Identification by the parents of the care the child will require after discharge
- ☐ Verbalization by the parents of reduced anxiety about the surgical procedure and follow-up care

Key interventions

- Reinforce the surgeon's explanation of surgery.
- Provide a tour of the pediatric facility, operating room, and recovery area. Show the child the staff's operating room attire, such as masks and gowns; allow the child to handle the anesthesia mask; tour the recovery room, discussing how long the child is likely to be there; and tour the waiting area where the parents will wait for the child during the surgery.

- Explain the preoperative routine to the parents and, in a developmentally appropriate manner, to the child. Explain that the child must have nothing to eat or drink before surgery; that surgery must be postponed if the child has a fever or cold symptoms on the day of the surgery; that the child will travel to the operating room in the parents' arms, if an infant, or on a stretcher, if older; and that oral or injectable preoperative medication will be administered. Also describe any laboratory tests that must be administered.
- Explain the typical postoperative care.
- Place the child on the side or in a prone position immediately after surgery.
- Record the characteristics of the ear drainage that usually is present immediately after surgery, and clean any drainage from the external ear.
- Provide clear liquids, progressing to a regular diet when full liquids are tolerated.
- Take vital signs every 15 minutes for the 1st hour after surgery and then every 30 minutes for the next 4 hours. When vital signs stabilize, the child will be discharged.
- Teach the parents the appropriate home care, including avoiding getting water in the child's ears by banning swimming and using earplugs during baths and shampoos for about 6 months; giving the full course of the prescribed antibiotic; giving acetaminophen as prescribed for pain and avoiding aspirin, which prolongs bleeding; reporting to the surgeon ear drainage that is bright red or occurs 3 days or more after surgery; reporting to the surgeon fever during the 1st week after surgery and thereafter reporting fever to the primary care practitioner; and reporting extreme pain to the primary care practitioner.

- Show the parents what the tubes look like. Explain that within 6 months, the tubes usually slip out and appear on the child's pillow. Advise the parents that this is not an emergency but that they should notify the primary care practitioner.
- Discourage nose blowing and hard coughing during the first 2 weeks after surgery because these activities may dislodge the tubes.
- Explain that some hearing loss may be evident during the first few weeks after surgery, and advise the parents to face the child and enunciate clearly when speaking.
- Have the child wear a cap or earmuffs in cold weather.

Otitis media

Inflammation of the middle ear.

NURSING DIAGNOSIS

High risk for injury related to lack of parental knowledge about otitis media

DESIRED PATIENT OUTCOME

The child will experience no permanent ear injury

Outcome measurement criteria

☐ Completion of a full course of the prescribed antibiotic

☐ Use of measures to prevent future inflammation of the middle ear

☐ Absence of signs and symptoms of ear infection

☐ Hearing within normal range

Key interventions

- Teach the parents the importance of administering the full course of the prescribed antibiotic.
- Advise the parents to consult the primary care practitioner if a rash or diarrhea develops while the child is taking the antibiotic.
- Teach the parents ways to prevent inflammation and infection, such as having the child wear earplugs while swimming, teaching the child not to put foreign objects or fingers into the ear, providing prompt care for suspected ear infections, holding the child upright when feeding, using a washcloth to clean the external ear, and never inserting cotton-tipped applicators into the ear canal.

- Teach the parents the common signs and symptoms of ear infection, such as fever, irritability, crying, and pulling on or rubbing the ear.
- Teach the parents how to control fever and make the child more comfortable, such as using acetaminophen as prescribed by the primary care practitioner; applying cool, moist washcloths to the child's face and arms; and placing minimal clothing on the child.
- Encourage the parents to take the child who has frequent ear infections to the primary care practitioner for a hearing evaluation.

NURSING DIAGNOSIS

Pain related to pressure secondary to ear inflammation or infection

DESIRED PATIENT OUTCOME

The child will experience relief from ear pain

Outcome measurement criteria

☐ Absence of indications of pain

☐ Peaceful sleep

☐ Relaxed appearance

Key interventions

- Administer an analgesic or antibiotic as prescribed.
- Apply heat by placing a warm cloth on the pillow and placing the affected ear on the cloth. Do not use a heating pad because it may injure the child.
- Use an ice compress to relieve pain if the child indicates that an ice compress reduces the pain.
- Remove ear drainage, using a warm washcloth.
- Assess the child's behavior after pain relief measures.

Tonsillectomy or adenoidectomy

Surgical removal of tonsils, pharyngeal adenoids, or both.

NURSING DIAGNOSIS

Anxiety related to lack of knowledge about the surgical procedure and postoperative care

DESIRED PATIENT OUTCOME

The parents and child (if age-appropriate) will demonstrate increased knowledge and reduced anxiety about the surgery and postoperative care

Outcome measurement criteria

- ☐ Verbalization by the parents and child (if age-appropriate) of the basics of the surgical procedure and the possible postoperative complications
- ☐ Verbalization by the parents and child (if age-appropriate) of the preoperative routine
- ☐ Participation by the parents in immediate postoperative care
- ☐ Identification by the parents of the care the child will require after discharge
- ☐ Expressions by the parents and child (if age-appropriate) of less anxiety about the surgical procedure and follow-up care

Key interventions

- Reinforce the surgeon's explanation of the surgery and its possible complications.

- Provide a tour of the pediatric facility, operating room, and recovery area. Show the child the staff's operating room attire, such as masks and gowns; allow the child to handle the anesthesia mask; tour the recovery room, discussing how long the child is likely to be there; and tour the waiting area where the parents will wait for the child during the surgery.
- Explain the preoperative routine to the parents and, in a developmentally appropriate manner, to the child. Explain that the child will travel to the operating room in the parents' arms, if an infant, or on a stretcher, if older, and that oral or injectable preoperative medication will be administered. Describe any laboratory tests that must be administered.
- Explain to the parents and child (if age-appropriate) the details of postoperative care.
- After surgery, place the child on the side or in a prone position.
- Maintain the I.V. line when the child returns from surgery, discontinuing it when the child is retaining liquids.
- Feed the child clear liquids, then full liquids, and then a soft diet.
- Give oral pain medication, as prescribed, for a sore throat.
- Apply an ice collar for 15 minutes every 3 to 4 hours on the 1st day.
- Measure vital signs every 15 minutes for 1 hour, then each hour for the first 6 hours, then every 2 hours for the next 6 hours, and every 4 hours thereafter.
- Check frequently for excessive swallowing or bright red secretions from the mouth or in vomitus.
- Explain to the parents that the child must urinate before being discharged. Before discharge, teach the parents appropriate home care measures.

- Warn the parents that the child is especially vulnerable to bleeding 7 to 10 days after surgery and that they should be alert for signs of bleeding, such as excessive swallowing, bright red secretions or vomitus, rapid pulse rate, and weakness, and should report them immediately to the surgeon.
- Advise the parents to control throat pain by giving acetaminophen every 6 hours as needed, to control ear pain with acetaminophen during the first 2 to 3 days after surgery and to report ear pain that persists for more than 3 days after surgery, to avoid aspirin because it prolongs bleeding, and to report increased throat pain or earache accompanied by fever.
- Tell the parents to encourage liquids and a soft diet for 3 weeks after surgery, to avoid hard or spicy foods, and to avoid using a drinking straw during the first few days after surgery.
- Tell the parents to discourage the child from coughing or blowing the nose hard during the first few weeks after surgery.
- Advise the parents that the child may return to school 1 week after surgery if no complications occur, but that they must provide for a soft diet at school and restrict strenuous physical activity until 3 weeks after surgery.

Appendicitis, acute

Inflammation or rupture of the appendix, which is treated with surgical removal of the appendix.

NURSING DIAGNOSIS

Anxiety related to lack of knowledge about preoperative procedures for appendectomy

DESIRED PATIENT OUTCOME

The parents and child (if age-appropriate) will demonstrate increased knowledge and reduced anxiety about preoperative procedures

Outcome measurement criteria

- ☐ Verbalization by the parents and child (if age-appropriate) of an understanding of appendicitis and appendectomy
- ☐ Statement by the parents and child (if age-appropriate) of why the child must not eat or drink before surgery
- ☐ Verbalization by the parents and child (if age-appropriate) of various routine preoperative procedures
- ☐ Demonstration by the parents and child (if age-appropriate) of reduced anxiety about the surgical procedure

Key interventions

- Reinforce to the parents the surgeon's explanation of the pathology of appendicitis and the surgery required to remove the appendix.

- Obtain a history of the present illness episode, including the occurrence of pain, nausea, and vomiting and the length of time between when symptoms first occurred and when assistance was sought from the primary care practitioner.
- Explain to the parents that pain medication may not be given until a diagnosis of appendicitis is confirmed because it may mask symptoms.
- Explain to the parents that to reduce the likelihood of aspiration during surgery, the child must not eat or drink after the time specified.
- Have the child empty the bladder before receiving preoperative medication.
- Explain preoperative medication (oral or injectable) to the parents and, in a developmentally appropriate manner, to the child.
- Explain that after the operation, the child will be returned to the room and will have an I.V. line in place.
- Dress the child in a hospital gown.
- Assess and record vital signs.
- Assess routine laboratory test results.
- Notify the surgeon of vital signs and laboratory test results not within normal ranges.
- Encourage the parents and child (if age-appropriate) to express concerns and fears; correct any misconceptions.

NURSING DIAGNOSIS

Pain related to inflammation secondary to incision for appendectomy

DESIRED PATIENT OUTCOME

The child will experience pain reduction to a tolerable level

Outcome measurement criteria

- ☐ Verbalization by the child (if age-appropriate) of reduced pain
- ☐ Demonstration by the child by sleeping or resting quietly that pain is absent or tolerable
- ☐ Absence of crying
- ☐ Relaxation of face and body
- ☐ Maintenance of normal ranges for pulse rate, blood pressure, and respiratory rate
- ☐ Ability of the child to tolerate movement and ambulation
- ☐ Resumption by the child (if age-appropriate) of self-care activities and social interactions

Key interventions

- Obtain from the parents a history of the types of pain previously experienced by the child and successful coping techniques.
- If developmentally appropriate for the child, assess the amount of pain using the children's pain scale.
- Administer prescribed medication regularly during the first 2 days after surgery.
- Use nonpharmacologic techniques to reduce pain, such as repositioning, relaxation, guided imagery, and distraction.
- Assess and document the child's response to medication and to nonpharmacologic pain-relief techniques.
- Monitor pulse rate, respiratory rate, and blood pressure every 4 hours. If they are below age-appropriate limits, withhold pain medication and notify the surgeon; if they are elevated, assess whether pain is being controlled adequately.
- Gently assist the child in moving carefully.

- Teach the child (if age-appropriate) how to splint the incision site with a pillow when turning and deep-breathing.
- Ambulate the child (if age-appropriate) as soon as prescribed. Initially, allow the child to ambulate only when the nurse or a parent is present to assist.
- Encourage a parent to stay with the child as much as possible.
- Plan care so that the child has periods of uninterrupted rest.
- Encourage the child (if age-appropriate) to participate in self-care activities and social interactions.

NURSING DIAGNOSIS

High risk for infection related to disruption of skin integrity by the incision

DESIRED PATIENT OUTCOME

The child will remain free from infection

Outcome measurement criteria

- ☐ Temperature below 100° F (37.8° C) for the first few days after surgery and below 99° F (37.2° C) thereafter
- ☐ Clear lung sounds
- ☐ Verbalization by the parents of potential sources of infection
- ☐ Demonstration by the parents and child (if age-appropriate) of good hand-washing technique
- ☐ Incision that is healing, pink, and approximated, with no signs of inflammation or purulence

Key interventions

- Assess vital signs and auscultate the lungs every 4 hours.

- Teach the parents the importance of washing their hands before and after contact with the child.
- Dress the incision site using sterile technique.
- Keep the dressing dry. Give sponge baths until sutures are removed.
- Inspect the incision site for redness, additional tenderness, purulent drainage, and dehiscence. Obtain a wound culture if purulent drainage is present.
- Monitor the child's white blood cell count.
- Gently assess the child's abdomen.
- If infection develops in the child's abdomen, place the child in semi-Fowler's position; administer I.V. antibiotics as prescribed, explaining the medication and the need for the I.V. route; describe the amount and character of drainage from the Penrose drain; and change the dressing as needed.

NURSING DIAGNOSIS

Fluid volume deficit related to nausea, vomiting, or both

DESIRED PATIENT OUTCOME

The child will be retain an adequate amount of fluid

Outcome measurement criteria

☐ Absence of nausea and vomiting

☐ Age-appropriate pulse rate and blood pressure

☐ Balance of fluid intake and output

☐ Adequate urine output (minimum of 2 ml/kg/hr)

☐ Age-appropriate urine specific gravity

☐ Presence of bowel sounds

☐ Elastic skin turgor

☐ Moist mucous membranes

Key interventions

- Assess vital signs, including blood pressure, every 4 hours.
- Monitor I.V. fluids for appropriate amount.
- Document fluid intake and output. Check urine specific gravity whenever the child voids or every 4 hours until the child's fluid intake returns to normal.
- Determine the presence of bowel sounds before giving fluids orally. Encourage clear fluids in small amounts initially and then offer the prescribed diet.
- Teach the family and child (if age-appropriate) the importance of a balanced diet for healing.
- Assess skin turgor for elasticity and mucous membranes for moistness.

Biliary atresia

Absence or obstruction of the bile ducts, which, if uncorrected, leads to cirrhosis and necessitates a liver transplant. Surgical correction often is possible using the Kasai procedure, in which a part of the jejunum is used to form a duct to carry bile from the liver to the small intestine.

NURSING DIAGNOSIS

Anxiety (parental) related to lack of knowledge about biliary atresia and associated care

DESIRED PATIENT OUTCOME

The parents will demonstrate increased knowledge and reduced anxiety about the child's biliary atresia and associated care

Outcome measurement criteria

- ☐ Verbalization by the parents of an understanding of the child's physical problems, including the necessity for surgical correction and the possibility of a liver transplant if complete liver failure occurs
- ☐ Verbalization by the parents of feelings about the child's condition
- ☐ Verbalization by the parents of increased comfort with the intensive care and hospital environments and with routine procedures
- ☐ Participation by the parents in the child's hospital care, such as assisting with bathing and comforting
- ☐ Verbalization by the parents of appropriate home care for the child

Key interventions

- Reinforce the surgeon's explanation about the child's condition, clarifying and answering questions.
- Explain the purpose of each test and procedure.
- Encourage the parents to openly discuss feelings and fears with each other, support each other, and initiate discussions with the staff about their feelings, fears, and questions.
- Consistently provide the parents with accurate information about the child's condition.
- Orient the parents to the intensive care unit (ICU) and the children's unit before surgery.
- Reorient the parents when the child arrives in the ICU and in the children's unit.
- Explain that medication will be given before surgery to make the child sleepy and after surgery to keep the child comfortable.
- Show the parents the room in which they will wait during surgery.
- Explain visiting policies for various units in which the child will be placed.
- Allow the parents to stay with the child and to participate in care as much as possible.
- Describe to the parents the various metabolic functions of the liver, explaining that these functions must be monitored by taking the child to scheduled appointments at the health care facility.
- Teach the parents how to care for the enterostomy and surrounding skin.
- Instruct the parents to monitor the child for signs of complications of surgery, such as unexplained fever and jaundice, and to report these to the surgeon immediately.

NURSING DIAGNOSIS

Fluid volume deficit related to decreased absorption or excessive loss of nutrients

DESIRED PATIENT OUTCOME

The child will exhibit fluid and electrolyte balance

Outcome measurement criteria

- ☐ Age-appropriate fluid intake and output
- ☐ Urine output of at least 2 ml/kg/hr
- ☐ Age-appropriate urine specific gravity
- ☐ Moist mucous membranes
- ☐ Elastic skin turgor
- ☐ Vital signs within age-appropriate ranges
- ☐ Absence of vomiting or diarrhea
- ☐ Absence of edema or ascites
- ☐ Age-appropriate weight
- ☐ Intact, nonpruritic skin
- ☐ Absence of signs of infection

Key interventions

- Document fluid intake and output carefully.
- Record color and amount of urine.
- Record urine specific gravity every 4 hours.
- Assess mucous membranes for moistness.
- Assess skin turgor for elasticity.
- Monitor vital signs, including blood pressure.
- Record the amount of vomitus and diarrhea.
- Note blood in vomitus or stool, and record the color of the stool.
- Measure abdominal girth daily and document changes.

- Weigh the unclothed child daily at the same time, using the same scale.
- Assess the skin for lesions and jaundice, and administer medication, as prescribed, for pruritus.
- Administer prophylactic antibiotics as prescribed.
- Monitor for signs of infection.
- Monitor laboratory test values.
- Administer water-miscible vitamins as prescribed.
- Provide a special, high-calorie formula for infants with liver disease, gradually moving to a normal diet after surgery.

Esophageal atresia and tracheoesophageal fistula

A congenital abnormality in which the esophagus ends in a blind pouch and an abnormal connection exists between the trachea and esophagus.

NURSING DIAGNOSIS

High risk for aspiration related to buildup of secretions

DESIRED PATIENT OUTCOME

The child will not experience aspiration

Outcome measurement criteria

- ☐ Bilaterally clear lung sounds
- ☐ Temperature below 99° F (37.2° C)
- ☐ Absence of cyanosis, choking, or retraction
- ☐ Pulse and respiratory rates within age-appropriate limits

Key interventions

- Intermittently suction the esophageal pouch and oropharynx to prevent buildup of secretions. Note the color and amount of suctioned secretions.
- Place the child in semi-Fowler's position.
- Do not allow the child any formula or water by mouth.
- Check vital signs and auscultate lung fields every 30 minutes.
- Observe for dyspnea and cyanosis.

- Document fluid intake and output carefully; weigh diapers.
- Monitor I.V. fluids for appropriate amount.
- Check the I.V. site for inflammation and signs of infiltration.
- Administer I.V. antibiotics and monitor for adverse effects.
- Assist with X-rays and other diagnostic studies.

NURSING DIAGNOSIS

Anxiety (parental) related to the consequences of the child's surgery

DESIRED PATIENT OUTCOME

The parents will demonstrate increased knowledge and reduced anxiety about the child's surgery

Outcome measurement criteria

☐ Verbalization by the parents of an understanding of tests and surgical procedures

☐ Discussion by the parents with each other and with staff members about their fears

☐ Demonstration by the parents of mutual support, such as standing close, touching, and holding

☐ Verbalization by the parents of an understanding of the child's condition and progress

☐ Verbalization by the parents of increased comfort with the intensive care and hospital environments

☐ Participation by the parents in the child's care, such as comforting and assisting with bathing

Key interventions

- Reinforce for the parents the primary care practitioner's explanation about the child's altered anatomy and physiology and the need for surgical correction, clarifying information and answering questions.
- Encourage the parents to openly discuss their feelings and fears with each other, support each other, and initiate discussions with the staff about their feelings, fears, and questions.
- Consistently provide the parents with accurate information about the child's condition.
- Explain the purpose of each test and procedure.
- Orient the parents to the intensive care unit (ICU) and the children's unit before surgery.
- Reorient the parents when the child arrives in the ICU and in the children's unit.
- Explain that medication will be given before surgery to make the child sleepy and after surgery to keep the child comfortable.
- Show the parents the room where they will wait during surgery.
- Explain the visiting policies for the various units in which the child will be placed.
- State the approximate number of days the child will be in the hospital.
- Allow the parents to stay with the child and to participate in care as much as possible.

NURSING DIAGNOSIS

Ineffective breathing pattern related to the effects of surgery for esophageal atresia and tracheoesophageal fistula

DESIRED PATIENT OUTCOME

The child will demonstrate an effective breathing pattern

Outcome measurement criteria

- ☐ Chest tube drainage output of no more than 2 ml/kg/hr during the immediate postoperative period
- ☐ Lung reinflation evident on chest X-ray film
- ☐ Vital signs within age-appropriate ranges
- ☐ Clear breath sounds bilaterally
- ☐ Normal cardiac rhythm

Key interventions

- Explain to the parents all procedures and treatments.
- Check the chest drainage setup to ensure that the drainage tube is straight, tubing connections are taped, dressing is secured over the chest entry site, and drainage system unit is below the child's chest level and secured so it cannot be knocked over.
- Keep two clamps for each chest tube adjacent to the water-seal setup for emergency use.
- Measure chest tube drainage by marking the level and time on the collection chamber every 15 minutes in the immediate postoperative period, then every hour for 24 hours, and then every 4 hours, unless otherwise indicated.
- Record the color of chest tube drainage, notifying the surgeon if 3 ml/kg of bloody drainage occurs within 3 hours, indicating a 15% blood loss. Excessive amounts of drainage must be replaced.
- Check chest tubes for patency. If the surgeon orders, gently strip chest tubes as prescribed in the immediate postoperative period.

- Report immediately to the surgeon if the child experiences dyspnea, cyanosis, sudden changes in breath sounds, or a lack of breath sounds on the affected side; hyperresonance on chest percussion; or absence of chest tube drainage although chest tubes are patent.
- Premedicate the child, as prescribed, 30 minutes before removal of the chest tubes.
- Tell the parents that the child will experience pain during chest tube removal but that the pain will not last long.
- Assist with the chest X-ray.
- Monitor the child for respiratory distress after chest tube removal.
- Give pain medication 30 to 40 minutes before chest physiotherapy.
- Make sure that chest physiotherapy is completed on time.
- Evaluate the effects of chest physiotherapy.
- Monitor vital signs for indications of inadequate oxygenation. Report cyanosis or restlessness to the primary care practitioner.
- Monitor oxygenation by means of pulse oximetry.
- Auscultate and percuss over the lungs each time vital signs are taken.
- Assess for bilateral symmetry of chest movements.
- Assess cardiac activity by means of a monitor.
- Encourage the parents to participate in some aspects of care, such as comforting or turning.

NURSING DIAGNOSIS

Fluid volume deficit related to losses secondary to surgery for esophageal atresia and tracheoesophageal fistula

DESIRED PATIENT OUTCOME

The child will display adequate fluid volume

Outcome measurement criteria

- ☐ Elastic skin turgor
- ☐ Moist mucous membranes
- ☐ Flat but not depressed fontanel
- ☐ Warm arms and legs
- ☐ Vital signs within age-appropriate ranges
- ☐ Strong and equal peripheral pulses
- ☐ Capillary refill time of less than 2 seconds
- ☐ Dressings with minimal drainage
- ☐ Fluid intake and output balanced and within age-appropriate ranges
- ☐ Urine output of at least 2 ml/kg/hr
- ☐ Urine specific gravity within age-appropriate range
- ☐ Electrolyte values within normal range

Key interventions

- Assess skin turgor, mucous membranes, and fontanel every 8 hours.
- Assess arms and legs for skin temperature.
- Monitor vital signs for indications of internal bleeding.
- Assess peripheral pulses, which should be strong and equal.
- Assess fingernails and toenails for capillary refill.
- Check the surgical dressing for drainage.
- Document fluid intake and output carefully.
- Check urine output every hour.
- Monitor urine specific gravity every 2 hours until the child's intake returns to normal.

- Monitor the I.V. fluid to ensure that the prescribed amount is infused on time.
- Monitor the I.V. infusion site.
- Weigh the child every 8 hours.
- Monitor serum electrolyte levels, especially the potassium level.

NURSING DIAGNOSIS

Altered nutrition: less than body requirements, related to an alternative feeding method secondary to gastrostomy

DESIRED PATIENT OUTCOME

The child will obtain adequate nutrition

Outcome measurement criteria

- ☐ Electrolyte levels within normal ranges
- ☐ Weight gain of 1 oz (28 g) per day, if medically appropriate
- ☐ Intact skin surrounding esophagostomy and gastrostomy
- ☐ Intake and output balanced and within age-appropriate ranges
- ☐ Absence of abdominal distention

Key interventions

- Monitor serum electrolyte levels.
- Weigh the child daily.
- Offer the child a pacifier during gastrostomy feeding.
- Leave the gastrostomy tube unclamped and draining to gravity until bowel sounds return. Then leave the tube open and elevated above the stomach level to allow air to escape.

- Give the first gastrostomy feeding after bowel sounds resume. Begin with clear liquids, gradually increasing to half-strength and then full-strength formula.
- Give feedings slowly and at room temperature.
- Assess the skin around the gastrostomy and keep it clean.
- Monitor the amount of drainage from the esophagostomy.
- Protect the skin around the esophagostomy and keep it clean.
- Change the esophagostomy dressing and bib as needed.
- Provide sham feedings to the older child during gastrostomy feeding.
- Maintain careful intake and output records.
- Monitor for abdominal distention.
- Encourage the parents to participate in some aspects of care.

NURSING DIAGNOSIS

Pain related to tissue trauma secondary to surgery and hospitalization

DESIRED PATIENT OUTCOME

The child will display signs of reduced pain

Outcome measurement criteria

- ☐ Verbalization by the parents of feelings about the child's painful procedures and treatments
- ☐ Demonstration by the child of increased comfort through relaxed posture, body movements, sleeping, and absence of crying
- ☐ Choices by the parents of measures that increase the child's comfort

Key interventions

- Encourage the parents to express feelings about the child's pain.
- Anticipate pain and institute pain-relief measures before its onset.
- Monitor the child's reaction to pain and note effective pain-relief measures.
- Give the parents an opportunity to assist in determining which measures decrease pain and increase comfort.

NURSING DIAGNOSIS

High risk for aspiration related to lack of knowledge about possible occlusion of the esophagus after surgical repair

DESIRED PATIENT OUTCOME

The child will not aspirate during feedings

Outcome measurement criteria

- ☐ Absence of aspiration
- ☐ Absence of choking or vomiting
- ☐ Absence of pain associated with swallowing
- ☐ Age-appropriate weight gain

Key interventions

- Feed the child in an upright position.
- Give formula or food slowly and in small amounts.
- Burp the child frequently during feedings.
- Note how feedings are tolerated.
- Stop the feeding and notify the surgeon if gagging, choking, or vomiting occurs.
- Stop the feeding if swallowing food causes the child pain or significantly changes vital signs.

- Prepare the child for esophageal dilatation, if necessary.
- Teach the parents feeding techniques and signs of esophageal occlusion.
- Weigh the child weekly at home and during scheduled follow-up visits.

Hepatitis

Inflammation of the liver, usually from a viral infection, such as hepatitis A virus (HAV) or hepatitis B virus (HBV). HAV is transmitted primarily by the GI route; HBV, by blood or blood-containing substances.

NURSING DIAGNOSIS

Altered nutrition: less than body requirements, related to anorexia, loss of GI secretions, or malabsorption

DESIRED PATIENT OUTCOME

The child will obtain adequate nutritional intake

Outcome measurement criteria

- ☐ Return to preillness weight
- ☐ Intake of age-appropriate, balanced diet and adequate fluids
- ☐ Stools, urine, and skin color that appear normal
- ☐ Urine output within normal limits (1 to 2 ml/kg/hr)

Key interventions

- Instruct the parents to weigh the child weekly.
- Advise the parents to report to the primary care practitioner if the child does not eat or drink satisfactorily.
- Teach the parents ways to increase the child's intake. Tell them to encourage the child to drink flavored oral replacement solutions; to stimulate eating by involving the child in food selection and offering attractive and interesting foods, if age-appropriate; and to encourage the child to eat low-fat foods, which are absorbed better.

- Teach the parents to keep intake (fluids and food) and output (urine and stool) records.
- Instruct the parents to observe the color and characteristics of the child's stool and to report clay-colored stool to the primary care practitioner.
- Instruct the parents to observe the color of the child's urine and skin and to report dark urine and yellow skin to the primary care practitioner.
- Advise the parents to report to the primary care practitioner if the child is lethargic, complains of dizziness, or behaves inappropriately.

NURSING DIAGNOSIS

High risk for infection (in others) related to lack of knowledge about hepatitis

DESIRED PATIENT OUTCOME

The child will not transmit hepatitis to others

Outcome measurement criteria

- ☐ Verbalization by the parents and child (if age-appropriate) of the mode of transmission for hepatitis
- ☐ Verbalization by the parents and child (if age-appropriate) of the time period during which the child's hepatitis is communicable
- ☐ Use of strict hand-washing techniques by the child (if age-appropriate), parents, and anyone else having direct contact with the child
- ☐ Use by the parents and other caregivers of universal precautions in handling body secretions or substances contaminated by body secretions
- ☐ Verbalization by the parents of the need for follow-up care to determine whether the child's hepatitis is still contagious and whether chronic hepatitis has developed

Key interventions

- Explain the mode of transmission and periods of communicability specific to the child's type of hepatitis.
- Teach the child (if age-appropriate) to wash hands appropriately and frequently.
- Teach the parents to wash hands appropriately before and after contact with the child; to properly dispose of body fluids and substances contaminated by body secretions; and to avoid sharing the child's toys with other children.
- Arrange for follow-up visits with the primary care practitioner to ascertain whether the child remains contagious and whether chronic hepatitis has developed.

NURSING DIAGNOSIS

Activity intolerance related to decreased energy

DESIRED PATIENT OUTCOME

The child will resume normal activities

Outcome measurement criteria

- ☐ Verbalization by the parents and child (if age-appropriate) of the relation between the disease and decreased energy
- ☐ Resumption of preillness activities
- ☐ Age-appropriate vital signs during activities

Key interventions

- Ask the parents about the child's activities before hepatitis occurred; use this information as a baseline for later activity assessments.
- Explain to the parents and child (if age-appropriate) why activity must be limited.

- Monitor the self-limiting of activity by the child and determine a rest schedule, if needed.
- Monitor vital signs during periods of activity if the child appears physically stressed.

NURSING DIAGNOSIS

High risk for injury related to medication ingestion during the acute stage of hepatitis

DESIRED PATIENT OUTCOME

The child will not experience injury caused by medication ingestion

Outcome measurement criteria

- ☐ Verbalization by the parents and child (if age-appropriate) of the dangers of giving medications during the acute stage of hepatitis
- ☐ Verbalization by the parents of the need to contact the primary care practitioner before giving any medications

Key interventions

- Explain how the liver functions, especially its role in metabolizing drugs.
- Discuss the importance of contacting the primary care practitioner before giving the child any medications, even over-the-counter drugs, such as acetaminophen and vitamins.

Hernia, inguinal or femoral

Protrusion of a loop of intestine into the inguinal or femoral canal.

NURSING DIAGNOSIS

Anxiety (parental) related to lack of knowledge about inguinal or femoral hernia and postoperative care

DESIRED PATIENT OUTCOME

The parents will demonstrate increased knowledge and reduced anxiety about the child's hernia and associated care

Outcome measurement criteria

- ☐ Identification by the parents of anatomic problems that may occur with an inguinal or a femoral hernia
- ☐ Verbalization by the parents of reasons why an inguinal or a femoral hernia should be repaired as soon as possible
- ☐ Statement by the parents of when emergency inguinal or femoral hernia surgery is necessary
- ☐ Verbalization by the parents of the details of routine postoperative care

Key interventions

- Explain to the parents and child (if age-appropriate) how an inguinal or a femoral hernia is created.
- Emphasize the importance of having a hernia repaired as soon as possible to reduce the risk of hernia strangulation or incarceration, which can lead to intestinal obstruction.

- Discuss methods to reduce the pain from a hernia, such as applying gentle pressure, comforting the child, placing the child in the supine position, or giving the child a warm bath.
- Describe the signs of hernia strangulation or incarceration, such as a persistent bulge in the inguinal area that cannot be reduced, fretfulness, crying, poor eating, difficulty with bowel movements, and abdominal distention.
- Teach the parents home care of the child who has undergone hernia repair, including giving prescribed pain medication every 6 hours for the first 48 hours and then observing the child's behavior to determine whether additional medication is needed; changing diapers twice as often as usual if the child is not toilet-trained and gently washing the diaper area around the incision; giving sponge baths instead of tub baths for the first 5 days after surgery or as prescribed by the surgeon; allowing the child to restrict personal activity; not permitting the older child to perform strenuous physical activity for 3 weeks; and notifying the surgeon if the incision becomes bright red, if its edges separate, or if purulence develops.

Liver transplant

Transfer and grafting of the entire liver or part of the liver from one person to another, most often performed on children when complete liver failure has occurred.

NURSING DIAGNOSIS

Ineffective family coping: compromised, related to uncertainty about a liver becoming available and the success of liver transplantation

DESIRED PATIENT OUTCOME

The parents and child (if age-appropriate) will cope with the uncertainty of the liver transplantation process

Outcome measurement criteria

- ☐ Verbalization by the parents of selection criteria for liver transplants
- ☐ Verbalization by the parents of an understanding of the transplantation process
- ☐ Use by the child of play therapy and pain-relief techniques
- ☐ Demonstration by the family of mutual support
- ☐ Identification by the parents of required care after liver transplantation

Key interventions

- Educate the parents about selection criteria for liver transplantation, explaining that the child must be free from infection outside the liver, cardiopulmonary disease, and human immunodeficiency virus infection and that the parents must be able to provide post-transplant care.

- Explain to the parents the aspects of preoperative child care, such as administering antibiotics, stool softeners, blood products, and diuretics; assessing the child's nutritional status; monitoring intake, output, and vital signs; describing changes in skin, stool, and urine color; and documenting bleeding episodes, including their location.
- Inform the parents about the tests and procedures that will be administered to prepare the child for transplantation.
- Use play therapy and pain-relief techniques to help the child cope with tests and procedures.
- Encourage the child and family members to express feelings openly.
- Encourage supportive actions within the family, such as kind words and deeds, hugging, and holding.
- Inform the parents about the intensive care measures that the child will require after the operation.
- Teach the family about the immunosuppressive drugs, such as cyclosporine and corticosteroids, that will be used after the operation, explaining that doses must never be missed.
- Educate the family about the signs and symptoms of organ rejection, such as tenderness over or enlargement of the liver, rapid pulse rate, elevated blood pressure, edema, and fever. Advise them to report any of these signs and symptoms to the primary care practitioner immediately.
- Caution the family about protecting the child from infection by avoiding people who are ill and large crowds and reporting signs or symptoms that may indicate the onset of infection.

Pyloric stenosis

A narrowing of the stomach's pylorus muscle that obstructs the flow of gastric contents into the small intestine and that can be corrected by surgery on the pyloric muscle.

NURSING DIAGNOSIS

Anxiety (parental) related to lack of knowledge about pyloric stenosis and pyloroplasty

DESIRED PATIENT OUTCOME

The parents will demonstrate increased knowledge and reduced anxiety about the child's pyloric stenosis and corrective surgery

Outcome measurement criteria

- ☐ Verbalization by the parents that indicates understanding of the child's condition and the need for surgery
- ☐ Identification by the parents of the usual preoperative and postoperative routines
- ☐ Verbalization by the parents of their questions and fears
- ☐ Demonstration by the parents of less anxious behavior

Key interventions

- Reinforce the surgeon's explanation of pyloric stenosis and corrective surgery.
- If the hypertrophied pylorus is palpable or visible as a bulge, explain the nature of the mass.
- Explain any visible peristaltic waves.
- Discuss X-rays and other diagnostic studies and specific preparation for them.
- Explain why preoperative I.V. therapy is necessary.

- Prepare the parents for the postoperative feeding routine.
- Encourage the parents to share their feelings and fears about surgery and other treatments.
- Give the parents a telephone number they can call to discuss questions or concerns before surgery.

NURSING DIAGNOSIS

Fluid volume deficit related to vomiting

DESIRED PATIENT OUTCOME

The child will display adequate hydration and normal electrolyte levels

Outcome measurement criteria

☐ Elastic skin turgor

☐ Flat but not depressed anterior fontanel

☐ Electrolyte levels within age-appropriate limits

☐ Serum pH within normal limits

☐ Vital signs within age-appropriate limits

☐ Absence of vomiting

☐ Balanced fluid intake and output

☐ Urine output of at least 2 ml/kg/hr

☐ Age-appropriate urine specific gravity

☐ Age-appropriate weight

Key interventions

- Assess skin turgor every 2 hours.
- Assess anterior fontanel for flatness.
- Monitor electrolyte levels and serum pH, notifying the primary care practitioner of levels outside the normal limits.

- Monitor vital signs every 2 hours, and monitor body temperature to detect hypothermia.
- Avoid giving the child anything by mouth, as prescribed by the surgeon.
- Note any vomiting, documenting the amount and character of vomitus.
- Monitor I.V. fluid intake to ensure that the child is not underhydrated or overhydrated.
- Check the I.V. site for signs of infiltration and infection.
- Provide a moistened pacifier as needed to comfort the child.
- Encourage the parents to hold the child, and carefully secure the I.V. line so the parents cannot accidentally dislodge it.
- Document fluid intake and output accurately, weighing diapers to ascertain output.
- Determine urine specific gravity every 2 hours.
- Weigh the child daily, noting weight decrease.

NURSING DIAGNOSIS

Altered nutrition: less than body requirements, related to the effects of surgery for pyloric stenosis

DESIRED PATIENT OUTCOME

The child will obtain adequate nutrition after the operation

Outcome measurement criteria

- ☐ Verbalization by the parents of comfort with feeding techniques
- ☐ Balanced intake and output
- ☐ Retention of feedings
- ☐ Absence of abdominal distention

- ☐ Return to age-appropriate weight

Key interventions

- Document the child's intake and output accurately.
- Administer I.V. fluids as prescribed and assess the need for hyperalimentation.
- Feed the child slowly and in an upright position, using a specific postoperative feeding schedule.
- Burp the child after feeding every 0.5 oz (14 g).
- After feeding, position the child upright or on the right side in an infant seat, or allow the parents to hold the child in that position.
- Note whether the child retains feedings.
- Teach the parents feeding techniques.
- Provide a pacifier as needed to comfort the child.
- Assess for abdominal distention.
- Measure abdominal girth immediately before surgery to obtain a baseline measurement. Measure girth every 4 hours after surgery if abdominal distention is noted.
- Withhold feeding and notify the surgeon if the child vomits a feeding or if abdominal distention occurs.
- Weigh the unclothed child daily at the same time using the same scale.

NURSING DIAGNOSIS

Pain related to inflammation secondary to surgical incision to correct pyloric stenosis

DESIRED PATIENT OUTCOME

The child will display signs of reduced pain

Outcome measurement criteria

- ☐ Relaxation of the child's face and body
- ☐ Demonstration by the child of the absence of pain through such actions as sleeping, resting, or lack of crying
- ☐ Pulse and respiratory rates within normal ranges
- ☐ Ability to tolerate movement

Key interventions

- Administer the prescribed medication regularly for the first 24 hours after surgery.
- Assess pulse and respiratory rates before giving pain medication. If rates are abnormally low, withhold medication and notify the primary care practitioner.
- Assess the amount of pain by observing the child's facial expression, body movement, and crying.
- Check the child for abdominal rigidity or distention every 4 hours, and notify the primary care practitioner if rigidity or distention is present.
- Ascertain the presence of bowel sounds every 4 hours, notifying the surgeon if sounds are not present.
- Move the child carefully and gently. Swaddle the child if the child seems more comfortable that way.
- Provide a moistened pacifier to comfort the child.
- Encourage the parents to hold the child in a way that ensures the child's comfort.
- Assess the child's reaction to medication and to positioning.
- Plan care so that the child has frequent periods of uninterrupted rest.
- Encourage the parents to remain at the child's side to soothe and comfort the child.

Vomiting or diarrhea

Signs of many disorders resulting from GI reactions. Vomiting is ejection of the contents of the stomach; diarrhea is an increase in the fluid content, frequency, and number of stools.

NURSING DIAGNOSIS

Fluid volume deficit related to increased loss of GI contents

DESIRED PATIENT OUTCOME

The child will display adequate fluid volume

Outcome measurement criteria

- ☐ Vital signs within age-appropriate limits
- ☐ Age-appropriate fluid intake
- ☐ Age-appropriate urine output (1 to 2 ml/kg/hr)
- ☐ Age-appropriate urine specific gravity
- ☐ Elastic skin turgor
- ☐ Flat but not depressed anterior fontanel, if patent
- ☐ Serum pH and electrolyte levels within normal limits
- ☐ Return to preillness weight
- ☐ Intact skin
- ☐ Verbalization by the parents of home care required

Key interventions

- Explain to the parents of the hospitalized child the need for various procedures and tests.
- Monitor vital signs every 4 hours.
- Document fluid intake and output accurately.

- Monitor I.V. fluids and the I.V. site.
- Encourage oral rehydration solutions if oral fluids are tolerated.
- Check urine specific gravity every 4 hours.
- Describe the characteristics and amount of diarrhea and vomitus, especially noting any blood.
- Check skin turgor every 4 hours.
- Palpate anterior fontanel every 4 hours.
- Monitor serum pH and electrolyte levels, notifying the primary care practitioner if they are not within normal ranges.
- Weigh the unclothed child daily at the same time and using the same scale.
- Clean the diaper area and apply a skin protectant.
- Note the child's behavior, such as irritability or lethargy.
- Question the parents if vomiting or diarrhea occurs after the child ingests certain foods or medications.
- Practice strict hand-washing technique and proper disposal of secretions.
- Teach the parents the appropriate home care, such as offering oral rehydration solutions in small amounts and gradually increasing the amount if fluids are tolerated; adding a bland diet without dairy products after clear fluids are fully tolerated; recording fluid intake and stool and urine output; noting the child's behavior; and notifying the primary care practitioner if vomiting or diarrhea does not stop, if fluid intake is less than appropriate for the child's age, or if fever develops.

General concerns related to hospitalization

Selected aspects of care that are encountered when a child is hospitalized and that apply regardless of the child's condition.

NURSING DIAGNOSIS

Anxiety related to the stresses of hospitalization

DESIRED PATIENT OUTCOME

The parents and child will display reduced anxiety about the child's hospitalization

Outcome measurement criteria

- ☐ Verbalization by the parents and child of decreased anxiety during hospitalization
- ☐ Use by the parents and child of effective coping techniques
- ☐ Demonstration by the parents and child (if age-appropriate) of the ability to focus attention on and to absorb explanations
- ☐ Open communication between the family and members of the health care team
- ☐ Resumption of appropriate eating and sleeping patterns by the parents and child
- ☐ Demonstration by the parents and child of relaxed behavior

Key interventions

- Assess the parents' and child's anxiety levels.
- Provide opportunities for the parents and child to express feelings and apprehensions and ask questions.
- Give the child opportunities to play through feelings or to draw pictures depicting feelings.
- Provide the parents and child with pertinent oral and written information, answering any questions they may have.
- Orient the family to the health care facility.
- Provide privacy for the family.
- Ask the family whether support people are available and, if so, whether the family wants these people present.
- Encourage family members to recall and use previously successful coping techniques.
- Assess the parents' and child's eating and sleeping patterns. Encourage the parents to eat regular, nutritious meals and to get adequate sleep; help the family create a system in which relatives or support people (if applicable) take turns staying with the child; and encourage the child to follow an eating and sleeping routine as much as possible while hospitalized.
- Use a play therapist, social worker, or psychiatrist, as needed, to assist the parents and child.

NURSING DIAGNOSIS

Anxiety related to lack of knowledge about procedures

DESIRED PATIENT OUTCOME

The parents and child will display increased knowledge and reduced anxiety about procedures

Outcome measurement criteria

- ☐ Verbalization by the parents and child (if age-appropriate) of decreased anxiety about procedures
- ☐ Identification by the parents and child (if age-appropriate) of the purposes of procedures
- ☐ Description by the parents and child (if age-appropriate) of what will occur during procedures
- ☐ Identification by the parents and child (if age-appropriate) of the preparations necessary for procedures
- ☐ Verbalization by the parents and child (if age-appropriate) of the knowledge that medication will be administered, if necessary, to keep the child as comfortable as possible
- ☐ Demonstration by the child of age-appropriate techniques to reduce anxiety and pain
- ☐ Signs of reduced anxiety, such as smiling, talkative child

Key interventions

- Assess the parents' and child's anxiety levels.
- Determine the parents' and child's previous experiences with this or other procedures.
- Explain the procedure's purpose and length, describing what will occur during the procedure.
- Let the child handle the equipment for the procedure, if possible.
- Show the parents and child where the procedure will be performed and where the parents will wait.
- Using age-appropriate language, explain to the parents and child the preparation for the procedure, including any injections, fasting, or enemas. For a young child, provide a concise explanation just before the procedure to avoid frightening the child or prolonging the child's anxiety.

- Assure the parents and child that anesthesia and analgesia will be used as needed to keep the child as comfortable as possible during the procedure.
- Teach the child age-appropriate methods of anxiety and pain reduction, including imagery and relaxation techniques.

NURSING DIAGNOSIS

High risk for ineffective family coping related to the effects of the child's hospitalization

DESIRED PATIENT OUTCOME

The family will cope effectively with the child's hospitalization

Outcome measurement criteria

- ☐ Verbalization by the parents of concerns, fears, guilt, and anger
- ☐ Identification of stressors
- ☐ Use by the parents and child of effective coping techniques
- ☐ Demonstration by family members of support for the child and one another
- ☐ Use by the family of support people or groups, social workers, and community agencies

Key interventions

- Encourage family members to express concerns, fears, guilt, and anger about the child's problems and to identify stressors.
- Ask family members to discuss the meaning of the child's illness to them, encouraging honest communication.

- Encourage the family to recall and use previously successful coping techniques.
- Promote the family members' self-esteem by recognizing and acknowledging effective coping efforts.
- Discuss the child's needs and ways in which family members can assist the child and staff in meeting those needs.
- Encourage family members to spend as much time as possible with the child, to participate in the child's care, and to offer one another periods of rest, away from the child and the situation.
- Encourage expressions of love and closeness between family members and the child.
- Contact the appropriate support people and groups, if the family desires, and refer the family to a social worker for help in obtaining financial aid and locating community support systems.

NURSING DIAGNOSIS

High risk for pain related to hospitalization experiences

DESIRED PATIENT OUTCOME

The child will display minimal discomfort

Outcome measurement criteria

- ☐ Verbalization by the parents and child (if age-appropriate) of feelings about painful procedures and treatments
- ☐ Choices by the child (if age-appropriate) of measures that increase comfort
- ☐ Verbalization by the child (if age-appropriate) of increased comfort
- ☐ Demonstration of the child's increased comfort on the age-appropriate children's pain scale

- ☐ Demonstration by the child of increased comfort through smiling, talking, and playing
- ☐ Relaxed posture of the child

Key interventions

- Encourage the family and child (if age-appropriate) to express feelings about painful procedures and treatments.
- Locate the pain site by asking the preschooler or older child to point to it.
- Assess the initial level of pain using the age-appropriate children's pain scale.
- Ask the parents about the child's usual reaction to pain and previously effective relief measures. Involve the parents in pain-relief measures, if possible.
- Teach the child age-appropriate pain-relief measures—such as controlled breathing, distraction games, heat or cold application, imagery, massage, music, pressure, relaxation techniques, and repositioning—to use in addition to medications.
- Allow the child (if age-appropriate) to tell the caregiver which measures increase comfort.
- Offer pain-relief measures 30 minutes before painful procedures, and assess their effects 30 minutes after administration, using the age-appropriate children's pain scale.
- Determine the most effective pain-relief measures for frequently performed painful procedures and treatments, and design pain-relief protocols for them.
- Provide opportunities for the child to play out painful experiences using dolls or hand puppets.
- Be truthful with the child about painful treatments and procedures, indicating about how much pain can be expected and how long it will last.

- Provide privacy during and after painful procedures and treatments to allow the child to regain composure.
- Allow the parents to be present during procedures and treatments if they wish and facility policy permits.
- Urge the child to remain still during painful procedures but to express pain, cry, yell, and squeeze the nurse's hand as needed. Praise the child for holding still during painful procedures.
- Encourage the parents to hold, comfort, and rock the child after painful procedures or treatments.
- Provide opportunities for the child to rest and enjoy uninterrupted sleep after painful experiences.

NURSING DIAGNOSIS

High risk for ineffective individual coping (child) related to the effects of hospitalization

DESIRED PATIENT OUTCOME

The child will cope effectively with hospitalization

Outcome measurement criteria

- ☐ Verbalization by the child (if age-appropriate) of feelings about hospitalization, treatments, and procedures
- ☐ Use of play to vent feelings and help the child understand and cope with procedures and tests
- ☐ Participation in play activities
- ☐ Signs of effective coping, such as smiling, talkative child

Key interventions

- Encourage the parents and child (if age-appropriate) to discuss feelings about hospitalization, treatments, and procedures.

- Provide opportunities for the child to play out procedures and treatments using dolls or hand puppets. Use these sessions to teach the child about upcoming procedures and treatments and to let the child vent feelings about past procedures and treatments.
- For infants ages 1 to 3 months, sing or play soft music; make frequent eye contact; provide a crib mobile; provide an active setting, if possible; call the infant by name; talk to, hold, and rock the infant; and play a tape of the parents' voices.
- For infants ages 4 to 6 months, provide soft, squeezable, or stuffed short-haired toys that are safely constructed; play soft music; talk to and laugh with the infant; call the infant by name; play a tape of the parents' voices; provide an unbreakable mirror in which the infant can see a reflection; provide larger toys that they can grasp, such as a rattle; and engage in bath splashing activities.
- For infants ages 7 to 9 months, play pat-a-cake or peekaboo; provide larger toys to prevent choking on toys or toy parts; provide teething toys; play the hunt-for-the-hidden-toy game; talk to and laugh with the infant; and play a tape of the parents' voices.
- For infants ages 10 to 12 months, read books and provide textured cloth books that the infant can handle; roll a ball to the infant, if feasible; show the infant how to build block towers; provide push-pull and other activity toys if the infant can use them; play music and sing; provide pans and a spoon; and talk to and laugh with the infant.
- For toddlers or preschoolers, play music and sing with the child; provide push-pull toys and fill-and-empty toys; read books; provide cloth books for toddlers and paper books for preschoolers; provide stuffed animals with secured small parts; provide large cardboard boxes, balls, pans, spoons, large-piece puzzles, dress-up clothing, and tools; talk to and laugh with the child; and play videotapes of siblings, if available.

- For school-age children, provide diversional activities, such as television, video games, books, music, artwork, and puzzles; provide building toys, such as model airplanes or cars; encourage puppet play and collections; and provide an opportunity to play with a pet, if possible.

NURSING DIAGNOSIS

High risk for injury related to an unfamiliar environment

DESIRED PATIENT OUTCOME

The child will not experience injuries due to hospitalization

Outcome measurement criteria

☐ Presence of name band on the child at all times

☐ Absence of medication errors

☐ Absence of aspiration

☐ Use of age-appropriate toys

☐ Closed exit doors in pediatric unit at all times

☐ Closed windows in pediatric unit at all times

☐ Use by the parents and child (if age-appropriate) of correct, consistent handwashing technique and appropriate protective gear

☐ Use of crib rails or side rails

☐ Absence of falls from cribs, beds, or stretchers

☐ Proper application of restraints

☐ Presence by the parents during the preschooler's or younger child's bath

☐ Behavior limits set by the parents for the child's protection

Key interventions

- Apply a name band to the preschooler's or older child's arm or the toddler's or infant's arm and leg; check daily for the presence of the name band; and carefully check the child's identity before performing procedures and administering medications.
- Perform procedures in a treatment room, keeping the child's room as a "safe space." If procedures such as drawing a blood specimen occur in the child's room, check the crib or bed carefully for small items that may have been left behind, such as a syringe cap, needle cover, or paper.
- Make sure that toys for a child up to preschool age are too large to be aspirated. Check toys for loose parts, poor construction, or small parts that the child can place in the mouth.
- Instruct the parents and visitors to keep the doors to the pediatric unit and the stairwells closed.
- Post instructions in the child's room advising parents and visitors to keep windows closed.
- Advise the parents to wash their hands frequently while staying with the child and to wear gloves if they have contact with contaminated fluids or secretions.
- Teach the parents to wear appropriate gear if the child requires isolation procedures.
- Teach the parents of an infant or a young child to keep up the crib rails whenever the child is not receiving direct care. Explain that when providing care in a crib, the parents must keep a hand on the infant at all times, especially if they must look away.
- Caution the parents of an older child to raise the bed's side rails when the child is sedated or sleeping.
- Place the bed in the position closest to the floor.

- Apply a restraint across the child's thighs before stretcher transport. Apply all restraints according to facility policy and the manufacturer's instructions.
- Advise the parents to stay with a child under age 6 during bathing.
- Ask the parents and the staff, when the parents are absent, to set limits to protect the child, such as prohibiting running in the halls or entering other children's rooms.

NURSING DIAGNOSIS

Sensory or perceptual alterations (visual, auditory) related to the hospitalization experience

DESIRED PATIENT OUTCOME

The child will demonstrate age-appropriate reactions to sensory or perceptual stimulation

Outcome measurement criteria

☐ Participation in age-appropriate play

☐ Appropriate interactions with others

☐ Alert, smiling child

☐ Age-appropriate sleep pattern

Key interventions

- Help the parents provide age-appropriate play activities for a child with sensory or perceptual deprivation. As the child's condition permits, encourage the child's friends, classmates, and relatives to send cards, telephone, and visit, if facility policy allows; encourage the parents to read or sing to the child and to accompany the child to a playroom or courtyard, up and down the hall, and elsewhere. Explain that the child may use a wheelchair or stretcher to leave the room or may be moved while in the bed.

- Organize nursing care to maximize rest for a child with sensory overload. Close the door to the child's room as much as possible; speak in a soft voice and move in an unhurried manner; program machinery alarms to sound at the nurses' station, if possible; play soft music to mask unit activity sounds; dim the lights in the child's room during sleeping hours; limit visitors; instruct visitors to talk softly and use minimal tactile stimulation; and give sedatives as prescribed to reestablish the child's sleep-wake cycle.

NURSING DIAGNOSIS

Anxiety (parental) related to lack of knowledge of the child's condition or care

DESIRED PATIENT OUTCOME

The parents and child will display increased knowledge and reduced anxiety about the child's condition and care

Outcome measurement criteria

- ☐ Verbalization by the parents and child (if age-appropriate) of an understanding of the condition's effects
- ☐ Verbalization by the parents and child (if age-appropriate) of the care required during the acute and chronic phases
- ☐ Demonstration by the parents and child (if age-appropriate) of the skills required for home care
- ☐ Participation by the parents in the child's care during hospitalization
- ☐ Identification by the parents of the child's actual, possible, and future needs
- ☐ Verbalization by the parents of community agencies available to provide assistance

- ☐ Statements by the parents and child (if age-appropriate) of decreased anxiety about the child's condition and care
- ☐ Verbalization by the parents of the child's need for anticipatory health promotion measures, such as dental care, immunizations, and a healthful diet

Key interventions

- Reinforce the primary care practitioner's and other staff members' explanations of the child's condition.
- Explain all care for the child's condition, using terms appropriate for the parents' educational level and the child's developmental level.
- Provide written information that the parents can refer to when providing home care.
- Demonstrate care, and ask the parents to demonstrate selected aspects of care.
- Encourage the parents and child (if age-appropriate) to participate in care during hospitalization and to assume increasing responsibility for aspects of home care, such as medication administration, suctioning, and dressing changes.
- Encourage the parents and child to ask questions about aspects of care that are unclear.
- Explain possible complications and future needs.
- Provide a list of resources that can assist the family.
- Stress the need for health promotion measures, such as immunizations, nutritious meals, adequate sleep, and regular dental care.

Cryptorchidism

Congenital undescended testicle.

NURSING DIAGNOSIS

Anxiety (parental) related to lack of knowledge about the child's condition

DESIRED PATIENT OUTCOME

The parents will display increased knowledge and reduced anxiety about the child's condition

Outcome measurement criteria

- ☐ Verbalization of knowledge about the child's condition and need for treatment
- ☐ Description of what will occur during surgery
- ☐ Identification of the expected outcome of surgery
- ☐ Verbalization of reduced anxiety about the child's condition and care

Key interventions

- Reinforce the primary care practitioner's explanation of the child's condition and the need for surgery, providing further information as questions arise.
- Explain the consequences if surgery is not performed, such as an abnormal-looking scrotum, related emotional trauma, an inability to be screened for testicular cancer, and probable infertility.

- Explain the surgery and its duration. Note that outpatient surgery is possible if the testicle is palpable and that brief hospitalization usually is necessary if the testicle is in the abdominal cavity.
- Explain that surgery should result in normal testicular appearance and adult testicular function.

NURSING DIAGNOSIS

Pain related to the effects of surgery to correct cryptorchidism

DESIRED PATIENT OUTCOME

The child will demonstrate signs of increased comfort

Outcome measurement criteria

- ☐ Lack of crying
- ☐ Peaceful sleep

Key interventions

- Administer an analgesic routinely, as prescribed, for the first 48 hours; thereafter, instruct the parents to give pain medication at the first sign of discomfort.
- Teach the parents to anticipate pain and recognize subtle signs of discomfort—disturbed sleep, restlessness, frowning, crying when moved, and poor eating—so that they can administer medication before pain becomes severe.
- Explain that medication will promote healing by keeping the child comfortable and allowing for adequate sleeping and eating.
- Instruct the parents to contact the primary care practitioner if the child's pain increases.

NURSING DIAGNOSIS

High risk for fluid volume deficit related to the effects of surgery to correct cryptorchidism

DESIRED PATIENT OUTCOME

The child will maintain age-appropriate fluid intake and output

Outcome measurement criteria

- ☐ Age-appropriate fluid and food intake
- ☐ Age-appropriate urine output
- ☐ Urine specific gravity within normal range
- ☐ Elastic skin turgor
- ☐ Soft, formed bowel movements

Key interventions

- Keep fluid intake and output records while the child is hospitalized, recognizing that adequate intake and output are required before the child is discharged.
- Check urine specific gravity at each voiding if fluid intake or urine output is inadequate.
- Check skin turgor.
- Instruct the parents to record the child's fluid and food intake and the number of wet-diaper changes and bowel movements during the first 3 days at home.
- Instruct the parents to contact the primary care practitioner if the child does not take and retain sufficient food and fluids, urinate adequately, or have soft bowel movements.

NURSING DIAGNOSIS

High risk for infection related to the effects of the surgical incision's location

DESIRED PATIENT OUTCOME

The child will display no signs or symptoms of infection

Outcome measurement criteria

- ☐ Intact, healed incision
- ☐ Absence of drainage or redness at incision site
- ☐ Absence of pain at incision site after initial healing
- ☐ Oral or tympanic temperature at or below 99° F (37.2° C); axillary temperature at or below 98° F (36.7° C)
- ☐ Age-appropriate fluid intake and urine output

Key interventions

- Protect the incision site with the prescribed dressing.
- Change the child's diaper frequently.
- Keep the incision site clean, immediately washing away any stool and changing the dressing as prescribed.
- Check the incision site for redness, drainage, and poor approximation of incision edges. Instruct the parents to observe daily for these problems and signs of incision pain after the initial postoperative period and to contact the primary care practitioner if problems develop.
- Take the child's temperature every 4 hours during hospitalization. Instruct the parents to take the child's temperature daily for the 1st week after surgery, notifying the primary care practitioner if the oral or tympanic temperature rises above 101° F (38.3° C) or if the axillary temperature rises above 100° F (37.8° C).
- Record intake, noting the child's ability to retain fluids during the immediate postoperative period; the child will be discharged when he or she consumes and retains fluids and produces adequate urine output. Instruct the parents to notify the primary care practitioner if the child refuses fluids and food or does not have adequate urine output.

Glomerulonephritis, acute

Inflammation of the glomeruli of the kidneys, usually preceded by a streptococcal infection.

NURSING DIAGNOSIS

Anxiety (parental) related to lack of knowledge about acute glomerulonephritis

DESIRED PATIENT OUTCOME

The parents will display increased knowledge and reduced anxiety about the child's condition

Outcome measurement criteria

- ☐ Verbalization of an understanding of the condition, its precipitating events, and its typical signs and symptoms
- ☐ Identification of possible complications
- ☐ Verbalization of an understanding of the necessary tests and procedures and the reasons for them
- ☐ Description of the continued care needed by the child after discharge
- ☐ Demonstration of decreased anxiety about the child's condition

Key interventions

- Reinforce the information about the condition provided by the primary care practitioner, offering additional information and explanations as needed.
- Give the parents written information about the child's condition, encouraging them to ask questions about the disorder, its usual signs and symptoms, and its possible complications.

- Assure the parents that the child is being monitored closely.
- Explain tests and procedures and their purposes, using age-appropriate language when speaking to the child.
- Discuss the home care the child will require, teaching about medications and procedures. Advise the parents to check the child's urine daily for blood and limit activity until urine is clear; to check the child's blood pressure daily, administering blood pressure medication as prescribed; to administer antibiotics as prescribed; and to protect the child from infection by practicing thorough handwashing and avoiding crowds and ill people. Teach the parents the importance of keeping follow-up appointments.
- Assess the parents' anxiety level periodically.

NURSING DIAGNOSIS

Fluid volume excess related to the effects of acute glomerulonephritis

DESIRED PATIENT OUTCOME

The child will display signs of normal fluid volume

Outcome measurement criteria

- ☐ Balanced fluid intake and urine output within age-appropriate ranges
- ☐ Yellow urine
- ☐ Urine specific gravity within age-appropriate range
- ☐ Return to pre-illness weight
- ☐ Absence of edema
- ☐ Intact skin
- ☐ Clear breath sounds
- ☐ Blood pressure within age-appropriate range

□ Oral or tympanic temperature at or below 99° F (37.2° C); axillary temperature at or below 98° F (36.7° C)

□ Absence of seizures

Key interventions

- Strictly monitor the child's fluid intake and urine output.
- Maintain the prescribed fluid intake, allocating specific amounts for meals, medications, and snacks if intake is restricted.
- Record urine color, noting changes from previous voidings.
- Check urine specific gravity at each voiding.
- Weigh the child daily.
- Check for edema, noting sites and amounts.
- Assess the skin for reddened or broken areas. Turn the child every 2 hours if the child does not move spontaneously, keep the skin dry and clean, and apply moisturizers as prescribed.
- Assess vital signs every 4 hours, noting crackles in lung fields and increased blood pressure or temperature.
- Administer diuretics and antihypertensives as prescribed to maintain blood pressure within the normal range.
- Monitor for headaches, visual disturbances, and other indications of hypertension.
- Take precautions to prevent injury if seizures result from elevated blood pressure.

NURSING DIAGNOSIS

Altered nutrition: less than body requirements, related to anorexia

DESIRED PATIENT OUTCOME

The child will consume an age-appropriate diet

Outcome measurement criteria

- ☐ Age-appropriate food intake
- ☐ Participation by the child in diet planning
- ☐ Age-appropriate weight gain

Key interventions

- Record the child's food intake.
- Provide a no salt–added diet, limit high-potassium foods if the child has oliguria, and restrict dietary protein, if prescribed.
- Encourage the child to choose from a list of appropriate foods.
- Provide foods that the child likes, and serve them in an appealing manner.
- Provide frequent, small meals rather than three large meals.
- Weigh the child regularly using the same scale and with the child wearing the same amount of clothing.

Hydrocele

Fluid in the inguinal or scrotal area, which may require surgery if it does not resolve spontaneously by age 1.

NURSING DIAGNOSIS

Anxiety (parental) related to lack of knowledge about hydrocele and related infant care

DESIRED PATIENT OUTCOME

The parents will display increased knowledge and reduced anxiety about the infant's condition and care

Outcome measurement criteria

- ☐ Verbalization of basic information about the condition and possible complications
- ☐ Verbalization of the need for surgery if hydrocele persists beyond infancy
- ☐ Identification of signs and symptoms that require the primary care practitioner's immediate attention

Key interventions

- Discuss the condition, informing the parents that if it persists beyond infancy, surgery may be needed.
- Encourage the parents to ask questions.
- Advise the parents that they will notice a bulge in the child's inguinal area, an enlarged scrotum, or both and that the scrotum may appear larger later in the day.
- Advise the parents to notify the primary care practitioner if the inguinal bulge becomes larger and the infant becomes fretful or cries, exhibits a distended abdomen, eats poorly, or does not have a bowel movement.

Hypospadias or epispadias

Congenital urethral malformations that usually occur in boys. In hypospadias, the urethra opens on the ventral side of the penis; in epispadias, on the dorsal side of the penis. Rarely, epispadias may occur in girls as a fissure in the urethra.

NURSING DIAGNOSIS

High risk for dysfunctional grieving (parental) related to loss of the infant's health

DESIRED PATIENT OUTCOME

The parents will cope effectively with grief associated with loss of the infant's health

Outcome measurement criteria

- ☐ Verbalization by the parents of an understanding of grieving
- ☐ Expressions of grief by the parents
- ☐ Verbalization by the parents of the effects of caring for an infant with hypospadias or epispadias on family life
- ☐ Verbalization by the parents of a plan to manage infant care initially
- ☐ Demonstration by family members of mutual support

Key interventions

- Assess the family's previous experiences with grief and loss, and determine if they successfully resolved the grief.
- Explain that grieving is normal, clarifying any misconceptions about grief.

- Encourage the parents to discuss their feelings about loss of the infant's health.
- Identify the strengths of the family unit and of individual members.
- Encourage the parents to be open and truthful with all family members.
- Prepare the parents for the possible reactions of people outside the family to the infant's condition.
- Discuss ways to manage the immediate details of caring for a sick infant, such as arranging care for other children in the family; making arrangements with employers; and modifying the home environment, as needed.
- Encourage the family to demonstrate mutual love and support.

NURSING DIAGNOSIS

Anxiety (parental) related to lack of knowledge about surgery for hypospadias or epispadias and related care

DESIRED PATIENT OUTCOME

The parents will display increased knowledge and reduced anxiety about the infant's surgery and related care

Outcome measurement criteria

- ☐ Verbalization of knowledge about hypospadias or epispadias and the eventual need for surgery
- ☐ Verbalization by the parents of the objectives of surgery
- ☐ Discussion between parents and staff about the parents' fears
- ☐ Verbalization of the home care needed by the infant before surgery

- ☐ Verbalization of the care the infant will receive immediately before and after surgery

Key interventions

- Reinforce the primary care practitioner's explanation of the infant's condition and the need for surgery.
- Explain to the parents that the objectives of urethral reconstruction are to make the penis appear and function normally and to make possible normal reproductive activity. Explain that accomplishing these objectives may require several surgeries.
- Explain that surgery is best performed before age 2 because after that age, the child is more likely to have castration or mutilation fears and, thus, be traumatized by genital surgery.
- Encourage the parents to support each other and discuss their feelings and fears openly.
- Encourage the parents to initiate discussions with staff members about their feelings, fears, and questions.
- Instruct the parents to protect the urethral mucosa, if exposed, by covering it with a prescribed moist gauze; to change the gauze with each diaper change; to change diapers frequently, thoroughly cleaning the diaper area after bowel movements to prevent irritation; to monitor for urinary tract infection by reporting to the primary care practitioner fever, dysuria, or redness around the open urinary tract; to provide for age-appropriate fluid intake; to notify the primary care practitioner if the infant is not consuming or retaining fluids.
- Orient the parents to the health care facility, including the pediatric unit and surgery waiting room.
- Explain that medication will be administered before surgery to promote sleep and after surgery to promote comfort.

- Explain the purposes of blood tests and preoperative procedures.
- State the approximate number of days the infant will be hospitalized.
- Allow the parents to stay with the infant and to participate in care as much as possible.
- Consistently provide the parents with accurate information about the infant's status.

NURSING DIAGNOSIS

High risk for injury (to the surgical site) related to activity after surgery

DESIRED PATIENT OUTCOME

The child will sustain no injury to the surgical site

Outcome measurement criteria

- ☐ Explanation by the parents of the purpose of the urinary drainage system that will be in place after surgery
- ☐ Verbalization by the parents of the importance of not moving the dressing or traumatizing the surgical site
- ☐ Demonstration by the parents of appropriate care for the urinary catheter or stent
- ☐ Identification by the parents of appropriate play activities for the child
- ☐ Verbalization by the parents of the need to keep the child well hydrated and free from infection
- ☐ Verbalization by the parents of the potential for psychological stress in the child who has genital surgery

Key interventions

- Avoid disturbing the surgical dressing. Be aware that the surgeon will perform the initial dressing change if a graft was used in reconstruction.
- Inform the parents that the catheter or stent drains urine from the bladder, maintaining the patency of the reconstructed urethra and allowing it to heal.
- Teach the parents how to irrigate the catheter, if prescribed, and show them how to keep the catheter or stent open and draining. Explain that the child will be discharged with the urinary catheter or stent in place and draining into the diaper or a collection bag.
- Use a bed cradle to keep bedcovers off the child. If needed, use arm and leg restraints or sedation to keep the child from traumatizing the surgical site.
- Release arm or leg restraints one at a time and exercise the restrained extremity every 2 hours.
- Encourage the parents to stay with the child to provide emotional support and a calming effect.
- Instruct the parents to keep the child's perineal area clean and to prohibit the child from engaging in play that is rough, potentially traumatizing, or likely to contaminate the surgical site.
- Teach the parents to keep the child well hydrated and to avoid situations in which the child may be exposed to infection.
- Explain that preschoolers typically have castration and mutilation fears and that genital surgery may be especially traumatic if the child is over age 2.

Kidney transplant

Replacement of a diseased, poorly functioning kidney with a donated one; considered an option when kidney failure necessitates dialysis and when families want to improve the child's quality of life.

NURSING DIAGNOSIS

Anxiety (parental, child) related to lack of knowledge about and preparation for kidney transplantation

DESIRED PATIENT OUTCOME

The parents and child will display increased knowledge and reduced anxiety about the transplantation

Outcome measurement criteria

□ Verbalization by the parents and child (if age-appropriate) of an understanding of the child's kidney problems

□ Description by the parents and child (if age-appropriate) of the advantages and possible complications of kidney transplantation

□ Identification by the parents and child (if age-appropriate) of the key measures before transplantation

□ Verbalization by the parents of feelings about the child's condition and impending surgery

Key interventions

- Reinforce the primary care practitioner's explanation about the child's kidney condition, answering questions and clarifying information.

- Explain that successful kidney transplantation negates the need for dialysis and certain dietary restrictions, allowing a more normal lifestyle. Inform the parents that transplantation also can result in rejection of the donated kidney and other complications, such as life-threatening infection.
- Explain the key measures necessary before transplantation, such as securing a donor, who can be a living person, such as a close relative, or someone who recently has died; clearing the child of all infection; and securing commitments from the parents and child (if age-appropriate) to the transplantation, regimen of care, and long-term medication.
- Encourage the parents and child (if age-appropriate) to express their feelings about a possible kidney transplant.

NURSING DIAGNOSIS

High risk for altered health maintenance related to insufficient knowledge about managing the treatment regimen

DESIRED PATIENT OUTCOME

The child will maintain health while recovering from kidney transplantation

Outcome measurement criteria

- ☐ Verbalization by the parents and child (if age-appropriate) of the prescribed treatment regimen
- ☐ Demonstration by the parents and child (if age-appropriate) of an accurate recording of food and fluid intake and output
- ☐ Demonstration by the parents and child (if age-appropriate) of correct techniques for testing the child's urine, stool, and blood and for checking the child's weight, blood pressure, and temperature

- ☐ Verbalization by the parents and child (if age-appropriate) of an understanding of the medication regimen, adverse effects, and risks of noncompliance
- ☐ Verbalization by the parents and child (if age-appropriate) of signs and symptoms to report to the primary care practitioner
- ☐ Verbalization by the parents and child (if age-appropriate) of the need for regular follow-up care by the primary care practitioner
- ☐ Verbalization by the parents and child (if age-appropriate) of their feelings about the child's condition and required care
- ☐ Use by the parents and child (if age-appropriate) of support groups

Key interventions

- Provide the parents and child with detailed instructions about the prescribed dietary regimen; monitoring food and fluid intake and urine output; testing urine for ketones, blood for glucose, and stool for occult blood; monitoring weight, blood pressure, and temperature; and recording all data.
- Describe the prescribed medication amounts and administration schedule, advising the parents to disguise the bitter taste by giving medications in syrup or jam or placing the medicine in a capsule, if the child is old enough to swallow one. Remind the parents to give an antacid with a prescribed corticosteroid.
- Teach the parents and child the usual adverse effects of immunosuppressant drugs, and warn them about the child's vulnerability to infection.
- Describe possible changes in the child's appearance caused by corticosteroid use, such as growth retardation, obesity, hirsutism, acne, and moon face. Discuss

ways to minimize these changes, and explain that they may diminish as the prescribed dosage is gradually decreased.

- Advise the parents and child about the dangers of discontinuing prescribed medications, such as transplant rejection (for immunosuppressants) and hypotension and shock (for corticosteroids).
- Emphasize that antirejection drugs must be taken for the remainder of the child's life.
- Alert the parents and child to signs of possible transplant rejection, such as continued lethargy, confusion, decreased urine output, increased blood pressure, and tenderness and edema over the transplant site. Advise the parents to report these signs immediately to the primary care practitioner.
- Instruct the parents to keep appointments with the primary care practitioner.
- Discuss feelings that the child may experience, such as guilt, stress, anger, and fear. Encourage the parents and child to discuss these feelings openly and honestly, and recommend that they become involved in a support group.

Nephrotic syndrome

Idiopathic disorder in which the glomerular membrane becomes permeable to protein, resulting in such problems as proteinuria, edema, and oliguria.

NURSING DIAGNOSIS

Fluid volume excess related to the effects of nephrotic syndrome

DESIRED PATIENT OUTCOME

The child will display normal fluid volume

Outcome measurement criteria

- ☐ Balanced fluid intake and urine output within age-appropriate ranges
- ☐ Yellow urine, free from protein
- ☐ Urine specific gravity within age-appropriate range
- ☐ Return to pre-illness weight
- ☐ Administration of corticosteroid medication as prescribed
- ☐ Absence of edema
- ☐ Intact skin
- ☐ Clear breath sounds
- ☐ Oral or tympanic temperature at or below 99° F (37.2° C); axillary temperature at or below 98° F (36.7° C)
- ☐ Age-appropriate vital signs, including blood pressure
- ☐ Absence of infection

Key interventions

- Strictly monitor fluid intake and urine output.

- Record urine color, amount of protein, and other abnormal urine characteristics, such as frothiness.
- Check urine specific gravity at each voiding.
- Weigh the child daily.
- Administer the prescribed corticosteroid accurately and consistently.
- Check for edema, assessing sites and amounts.
- Provide support for an edematous scrotum and elevate edematous arms and legs.
- Assess the skin for reddened or broken areas, turn the child every 2 hours if the child does not move spontaneously, and keep the skin dry and clean.
- Assess vital signs every 4 hours, especially noting crackles in lung fields and increased blood pressure or temperature.
- Encourage thorough, frequent handwashing by the child and caregivers, and avoid contact between the child and ill people.

NURSING DIAGNOSIS

Altered nutrition: less than body requirements, related to anorexia

DESIRED PATIENT OUTCOME

The child will consume an age-appropriate diet

Outcome measurement criteria

☐ Participation by the child in diet planning

☐ Intake of a low-sodium, high-protein diet

☐ Age-appropriate weight

Key interventions

- Encourage the child to choose from a list of appropriate foods, providing as many favorite foods as possible.
- Provide frequent, small meals rather than three large meals.
- Provide the prescribed low-sodium, high-protein diet, noting the amount taken, how it is tolerated, and the number of calories consumed.
- Weigh the child regularly.

NURSING DIAGNOSIS

Fatigue related to the effects of nephrotic syndrome

DESIRED PATIENT OUTCOME

The child will participate in activities without undue fatigue

Outcome measurement criteria

- ☐ Participation in quiet, age-appropriate play and activities
- ☐ Vital signs within normal limits

Key interventions

- Provide opportunities for age-appropriate games and activities that require minimal energy.
- Schedule rest periods.
- Organize nursing care so that rest and sleep periods are disturbed as little as possible.
- Assess the child's vital signs before and after activity. Monitor the child's reaction to activity.

NURSING DIAGNOSIS

High risk for infection related to the effects of nephrotic syndrome and its treatment

DESIRED PATIENT OUTCOME

The child will display no signs or symptoms of infection

Outcome measurement criteria

- ☐ Clear breath sounds
- ☐ Age-appropriate heart and respiratory rates
- ☐ Oral or tympanic temperature at or below 99° F (37.2° C); axillary temperature at or below 98° F (36.7° C)
- ☐ Age-appropriate white blood cell (WBC) count and erythrocyte sedimentation rate
- ☐ Intact skin and mucous membranes
- ☐ Use by the family of proper handwashing technique

Key interventions

- Auscultate lung fields, assess heart and respiratory rates, and check the temperature every 4 hours.
- Review test results for signs of infection, such as elevated WBC count and erythrocyte sedimentation rate.
- Turn the child every 2 hours if the child does not move spontaneously to help maintain skin integrity.
- Do not allow people who appear ill to visit the child.
- Use proper handwashing technique, and teach the family to wash hands thoroughly and frequently.

NURSING DIAGNOSIS

High risk for ineffective management of therapeutic regimen (parental) related to lack of knowledge about nephrotic syndrome and related home care

DESIRED PATIENT OUTCOME

The parents will display increased knowledge about the child's condition and home care

Outcome measurement criteria

- ☐ Statement of an understanding of nephrotic syndrome, its precipitating events, and its signs and symptoms
- ☐ Verbalization of possible complications
- ☐ Identification of reasons for tests and procedures
- ☐ Verbalization of necessary home care

Key interventions

- Provide written information about nephrotic syndrome and encourage the parents to ask questions about the syndrome and its usual signs and symptoms. Reinforce information given by the primary care practitioner about the syndrome and its possible complications.
- Explain to the parents and child (in an age-appropriate manner) all tests and procedures and their reasons.
- Discuss the child's home care needs, advising the parents to protect the child from infections, monitor for signs of infection, and make sure that they and the child use proper handwashing technique.
- Teach the parents to measure the child's blood pressure and weight daily.
- Teach the parents about the prescribed corticosteroid's usual adverse effects, dosage regimen, and duration of therapy. Advise them not to discontinue the drug until instructed.
- Emphasize the need for the child to attend scheduled follow-up appointments.

Ureteral reimplantation

Surgical removal and reattachment of the ureter to the bladder to correct a congenital urinary tract anomaly, prevent urine reflux, and promote urine drainage from the kidneys to the bladder.

NURSING DIAGNOSIS

Anxiety (parental, child) related to lack of knowledge about the child's condition and treatment

DESIRED PATIENT OUTCOME

The parents and child (if age-appropriate) will display increased knowledge and reduced anxiety about the child's condition and treatment

Outcome measurement criteria

- ☐ Verbalization by the parents and child (if age-appropriate) of knowledge about the child's condition and the need for treatment
- ☐ Verbalization by the parents and child (if age-appropriate) of what will occur during surgery
- ☐ Statements by the parents and child (if age-appropriate) of the expected outcome of surgery
- ☐ Verbalization by the parents and child (if age-appropriate) of decreased anxiety about the child's condition

Key interventions

- Reinforce the primary care practitioner's explanation of the child's condition and the need for surgery.

- Provide further explanations as questions arise, and offer information about complications that can occur if surgery is not performed, such as chronic urinary tract infections, kidney damage, and, possibly, kidney failure.
- Explain the surgical procedure using pictures and age-appropriate language. Estimate the surgery's duration, and explain that surgery will necessitate several days' hospitalization.
- Discuss that the anticipated result of surgery is normal bladder function.
- Assess the parents' anxiety level. Provide additional information and support as needed.

NURSING DIAGNOSIS

Pain related to the effects of the surgical incision and related procedures

DESIRED PATIENT OUTCOME

The child will display signs of increased comfort

Outcome measurement criteria

- ☐ Verbalization by the parents and child (if age-appropriate) of feelings about painful procedures and the incision
- ☐ Verbalization by the child (if age-appropriate) of increased comfort
- ☐ Demonstration by the child of increased comfort through smiling, talking, playing, and relaxed posture
- ☐ Demonstration of increased comfort on the age-appropriate children's pain scale
- ☐ Choices by the child (if age-appropriate) of measures that increase comfort

Key interventions

- Encourage the child and family to express feelings about the child's pain and incision.
- Ask the parents about the child's usual reaction to pain and effective relief measures. Involve the parents in pain-relief measures, if possible.
- Locate the pain site by asking the preschooler or older child to point to it.
- Assess the initial pain level using the age-appropriate children's pain scale.
- If age-appropriate, teach the child pain-relief measures to use in addition to medications, such as controlled breathing, distraction games, heat or cold application, imagery, massage, pressure, relaxation techniques, and repositioning.
- Anticipate pain, and offer analgesics, as prescribed, and pain-relief measures before pain becomes severe.
- Determine the effects of analgesics and other pain-relief measures 30 minutes after administration by using the age-appropriate children's pain scale. Be aware that an older child may use patient-controlled analgesia.
- Give the child (if age-appropriate) an opportunity to tell which measures decrease pain and increase comfort.
- Provide opportunities for the child to play out painful experiences using dolls or hand puppets.
- Be truthful with the child about painful treatments and procedures, indicating about how much pain can be expected and how long it will last.
- Provide privacy during and after procedures and treatments to allow the child to regain composure.
- Encourage the parents to be present during dressing changes and procedures.

- Encourage the child to remain still during procedures but to express pain, cry, yell, and squeeze the nurse's hand as needed. Reward the child for remaining still during painful procedures.
- Encourage the parents to hold, comfort, and rock the child after painful procedures or treatments.
- Provide opportunities for the child to rest and enjoy periods of uninterrupted sleep after painful experiences.

NURSING DIAGNOSIS

High risk for infection related to the surgical incision and urinary diversion devices

DESIRED PATIENT OUTCOME

The child will display no signs or symptoms of infection

Outcome measurement criteria

- ☐ Intact, healed incision
- ☐ Absence of redness at incision site
- ☐ Absence of purulence at the incision site and stent or catheter exit sites
- ☐ Clear, yellow urine
- ☐ Oral or tympanic temperature at or below 99° F (37.2° C); axillary temperature at or below 98° F (36.7° C)
- ☐ Compliance with the prescribed antibiotic regimen
- ☐ Age-appropriate food and fluid intake

Key interventions

- Protect the incision site with a dressing, changing and cleaning it as prescribed, using sterile technique.
- Observe the incision site for redness, drainage, and poor approximation of incision edges. Culture the site if purulence or other signs of infection are present.

- Protect stent exit sites with sterile dressings. Be aware that the surgeon may change these dressings.
- Monitor the drainage of stents into the urine collection device. Understand that gross hematuria occurs initially but that stent drainage gradually should become clear.
- Use an antimicrobial solution to clean around the catheter exit site at least every 8 hours. If the catheter exits through the urethra, clean more frequently. If it exits through the suprapubic area, change the dressing as prescribed, usually daily.
- Empty urine from stent and catheter collection devices using sterile technique. Record urine color and clarity and the amount of drainage, and obtain a urine specimen for culture if the child shows signs of urinary tract infection.
- Take the child's temperature every 4 hours, giving an antipyretic as prescribed if the oral or tympanic temperature rises above 101° F (38.3° C) or if the axillary temperature rises above 100° F (37.8° C). Recheck the temperature 1 hour after antipyretic administration, and record the response to the medication.
- Monitor the I.V. infusion rate, and observe the I.V. site for signs of infiltration, redness, or pain.
- Administer antibiotics as prescribed. Explain to the parents the need to give antibiotics consistently and to encourage the child to drink large quantities of fluids while receiving antibiotics.
- Record fluid intake, and note the child's ability to retain fluids as soon as bowel sounds are present and oral intake is prescribed. Encourage fluids and nutrients by providing favorite liquids and foods. Instruct the parents to notify the primary care practitioner if the child refuses fluids and food or does not have adequate urine output after discharge.

Acquired immunodeficiency syndrome

Fatal syndrome of viral origin in which the immune system becomes severely depressed, resulting in extreme susceptibility to life-threatening opportunistic infections and rare cancers.

NURSING DIAGNOSIS

Fear (parental, child) related to the effects of acquired immunodeficiency syndrome (AIDS) and its fatal prognosis

DESIRED PATIENT OUTCOME

The parents and child will display improved coping skills, reduced fear, and increased knowledge of the child's disease, including its probable course and outcome

Outcome measurement criteria

- ☐ Verbalization by the parents and child (if age-appropriate) of a basic understanding of AIDS
- ☐ Description by the parents and child (if age-appropriate) of the universal precautions to be used
- ☐ Sharing by the parents and child (if age-appropriate) of feelings about the child's disease
- ☐ Discussion by the parents of their feelings if either of them tests positive for the human immunodeficiency virus (HIV)
- ☐ Expression by the parents of feelings about the way in which the child acquired the disease

- ☐ Verbalization by the parents and child (if age-appropriate) of possible reactions to the diagnosis by family and friends
- ☐ Identification by the parents and child (if age-appropriate) of sources of support

Key interventions

- Discuss, in basic terms and over several counseling sessions, the pathophysiology of AIDS, encouraging the parents and child (if age-appropriate) to ask questions.
- Detail the universal precautions for handling body fluids outlined by the Centers for Disease Control and Prevention. Instruct the parents when to wear gloves and how to dispose of contaminated articles. Explain that casual and routine home contact will not result in HIV transmission to other family members.
- Openly discuss the parents' and child's feelings about the disease, such as anger, fear, anxiety, and hopelessness.
- Encourage the parents to express feelings about the way in which the child acquired the disease, whether from the mother at birth or during breast-feeding, through a blood transfusion, or from sexual abuse, I.V. drug abuse, or unprotected sexual activity.
- Discuss the possible reactions of family and friends to the child's AIDS. Teach ways to educate them about HIV transmission to reduce fear of contact with the child.
- Discuss sources of support, such as relatives and friends, AIDS support groups, the health care team, clergy members, and community agencies that assist AIDS patients.

NURSING DIAGNOSIS

High risk for infection related to a compromised immune system

DESIRED PATIENT OUTCOME

The child will display no signs or symptoms of infection

Outcome measurement criteria

- ☐ Age-appropriate food and fluid intake
- ☐ Oral temperature below 99° F (37.2° C)
- ☐ Clear breath sounds in all fields
- ☐ Absence of rashes, lesions, or purulent drainage
- ☐ Clear, yellow urine
- ☐ Absence of signs and symptoms of opportunistic infection
- ☐ Alert, active child

Key interventions

- Instruct the parents and child to use proper handwashing technique at home.
- Warn the parents to protect the child from obvious sources of infection, such as large crowds and ill people.
- Teach the parents to check for signs and symptoms of infection, such as anorexia, lethargy, coughing, congestion, wheezing, dyspnea, rashes, lesions, purulent drainage, and dysuria, and to report these to the primary care practitioner. Instruct them to take the child's temperature every 4 hours if they suspect infection and to report a rise in temperature to the primary care practitioner immediately; hospitalization may be necessary.
- Implement universal precautions if the child is hospitalized. Wear a gown, mask, and goggles if the child is bleeding heavily or has a productive cough; isolate the child to protect him or her from infectious organisms in the health care facility; and use sterile technique as appropriate.

- Document fluid intake and urine output during hospitalization, also noting urine clarity and color. Note diarrhea, and test stool for occult blood. Monitor the I.V. for the prescribed rate, and check the I.V. site for signs of infiltration or infection.
- Provide high-calorie fluids and foods the child likes.
- Administer I.V. antibiotics, gamma globulin, and other medications as prescribed, noting any reactions to medications.
- Take vital signs every 4 hours, and administer an antipyretic as prescribed if the oral temperature exceeds 101° F (38.3° C). Record the child's response to antipyretics, and take other fever-reduction measures, such as removing some of the child's clothing and bedcovers and lowering the room temperature.
- Carefully auscultate lungs, noting crackles and rhonchi and recording the degree of respiratory distress.
- Observe for rashes, lesions, and purulent drainage, describing them and noting their location.
- Review the results of laboratory tests, alerting the primary care practitioner to signs of infection.

NURSING DIAGNOSIS

High risk for altered health maintenance related to the complexity of the care regimen

DESIRED PATIENT OUTCOME

The parents will manage the child's care effectively

Outcome measurement criteria

- ☐ Verbalization by the parents, any siblings, and the child (if age-appropriate) of the need to use universal precautions when handling body secretions and disposing of wastes contaminated with blood and other body fluids

- ☐ Verbalization by the parents, any siblings, and the child (if age-appropriate) of the need to protect the child from infections
- ☐ School attendance by the child (if age-appropriate)
- ☐ Socialization by the child with other children
- ☐ Use by the family of community resources

Key interventions

- Discuss with family members and the child (if age-appropriate) the ways in which HIV is transmitted.
- Describe to the parents, any siblings, and the child (if age-appropriate) how to use universal precautions when handling body secretions.
- Develop a plan for disposing of wastes contaminated with blood or other body secretions.
- Discuss with the child, if an adolescent, the need for responsible sexual behavior.
- Explain to the parents, any siblings, and the child (if age-appropriate) that casual contact with the child does not transmit HIV.
- Describe ways to protect the child with AIDS from infections, including avoiding large crowds in close quarters, avoiding group contact during influenza and cold seasons, obtaining all prescribed immunizations, obtaining gamma globulin if prescribed by the primary care practitioner, and avoid people with obvious infections.
- Promote school attendance, if age-appropriate, by providing information for school personnel. Tell the parents they probably will need a statement from the primary care practitioner indicating that school attendance is appropriate. Ask the parents to meet with the school nurse and the child's teacher to explain special care that may be needed during the school day, such as

checking the child's activity level and treating nosebleeds or vomiting.

- Develop a plan for the child to use at school to handle contaminated items, such as bloody tissues or soiled sanitary napkins.
- Encourage the child to participate in school activities but to avoid contact sports.
- Prepare the family and child (if age-appropriate) for the possible negative responses by other people to the child with AIDS.
- Help the family obtain assistance and resources from community agencies and AIDS support groups.

Hemophilia A

Inherited, X-linked recessive disease that results in a deficiency or absence of coagulation factor VIII activity, causing various degrees of spontaneous bleeding, bleeding from trauma or surgery, or both.

NURSING DIAGNOSIS

Anxiety (parental) related to lack of knowledge about the child's condition

DESIRED PATIENT OUTCOME

The parents will display increased knowledge and reduced anxiety about the child's condition

Outcome measurement criteria

- ☐ Demonstration by the parents of a basic understanding of hemophilia A and the need for treatment
- ☐ Verbalization by the parents of the expected course of hemophilia A and its outcome, depending on the degree of factor VIII deficiency
- ☐ Expression by the parents of feelings about the child's inherited disease
- ☐ Verbalization by the parents of increased comfort with the child's condition

Key interventions

- Reinforce the primary care practitioner's explanation of the child's condition and the need to follow the prescribed treatment regimen, including replacement of factor VIII.
- Explain that the blood level of factor VIII will determine the severity of the child's signs and symptoms.

- Provide further information as questions arise. Also discuss the complications that can occur if the disease is not treated.
- Encourage the parents and child to express feelings about the child's inheritance of a serious disease.
- Refer the parents for genetic counseling.

NURSING DIAGNOSIS

High risk for altered health maintenance related to the effects of the child's newly diagnosed hemophilia A

DESIRED PATIENT OUTCOME

The child will experience a minimal number of bleeding episodes and no excessive bleeding

Outcome measurement criteria

☐ Wearing by the child of a medical identification bracelet

☐ Verbalization by the parents and child (if age-appropriate) of an understanding of the appropriate preventive and treatment regimen

☐ Demonstration by the parents and child (if age-appropriate) of an ability to manage the child's injuries

☐ Absence of excessive bleeding

☐ Bleeding time and factor VIII levels within normal limits

☐ Awareness by the child's teacher (if applicable) of the child's condition

☐ Participation by the child in age-appropriate play and activities

Key interventions

- Instruct the parents to have the child wear a medical identification bracelet.

- Teach the parents to modify the home environment to decrease the risk of bleeding injuries. Advise them to provide age-appropriate toys without sharp parts; to pad crib sides; to carpet floors; to use padded furniture as much as possible where the child plays; and to remove from the younger child objects that can cause injury, such as scissors, sharp tools, knives, and pins, and to supervise the older child's use of these objects.
- Teach the parents to have the child wear elbow and knee pads and a helmet, especially during play.
- Advise the parents to keep follow-up appointments to monitor the factor VIII level and bleeding time.
- Teach the parents how to care for injuries. For minor injuries, advise them to immobilize and elevate the injured area, apply pressure for 15 minutes, and apply ice. For major injuries, tell them to give recombinant factor VIII, apply ice, apply pressure for 15 minutes, immobilize and elevate the injured area above heart level, and seek medical assistance to monitor vital signs and blood pressure if the child is actively bleeding.
- Urge the parents to tell the child's teacher (if applicable) about the child's condition and to provide written information about first aid for injuries as well as telephone numbers where the parents can be reached.
- Encourage the parents and child to decide which activities are appropriate for the child. Advise them to avoid contact sports and to encourage such exercises as swimming and golfing, unless prohibited by joint damage.

NURSING DIAGNOSIS

Pain related to the effects of bleeding into tissues

DESIRED PATIENT OUTCOME

The child will display increased comfort

Outcome measurement criteria

- ☐ Verbalization by the child (if age-appropriate) of increased comfort
- ☐ Demonstration by the child of increased comfort on the age-appropriate children's pain scale
- ☐ Demonstration by the child of increased comfort through smiling, talking, and playing
- ☐ Verbalization by the parents and child (if age-appropriate) of feelings about painful bleeding episodes

Key interventions

- Provide immediate trauma treatment, including pressure, ice, immobilization, and elevation. If the injury is in a joint or a location that makes it difficult to apply pressure or ice, give factor VIII as prescribed. Administer corticosteroids if prescribed.
- Keep an injured joint immobilized and elevated until bleeding has stopped. Then provide range-of-motion exercises and physical therapy to minimize permanent disability.
- Assess the level of pain using the age-appropriate children's pain scale.
- Administer a nonaspirin analgesic, and assess pain relief 30 minutes after administration using the age-appropriate children's pain scale.
- Provide quiet diversional activities, such as reading, board games, and videos.
- Encourage the parents and child to express feelings about the child's painful episodes.
- Provide opportunities for the child to play out painful experiences using dolls or hand puppets.

Iron deficiency anemia

Subnormal hemoglobin level due to insufficient dietary iron intake.

NURSING DIAGNOSIS

Altered health maintenance related to lack of knowledge about appropriate dietary iron intake

DESIRED PATIENT OUTCOME

The child will consume an age-appropriate diet that contains sufficient iron to meet the body's needs

Outcome measurement criteria

- ☐ Verbalization by the parents of an understanding of the child's need for supplementary iron
- ☐ Age-appropriate diet
- ☐ Hemoglobin level within normal range
- ☐ Age-appropriate weight

Key interventions

- Educate the parents about anemia prevention. Provide dietary information to the parents of a full-term neonate during the 4-month visit, informing them that bottle-fed infants should receive iron-fortified formula and breast-fed infants should receive iron-fortified baby cereal. Provide dietary information to the parents of a breast-fed preterm neonate during the 2-month visit, informing them that the infant needs iron drops and, later, iron-fortified cereals. Advise the parents to limit the formula or milk intake of the child age 1 or older to 1 qt per day. Encourage the parents of an infant or toddler to feed solid foods before providing formula for an infant or milk for a toddler. Instruct the parents to limit the child's intake of iron-poor foods, such as sweets and starches. Encourage weaning the child from the bottle by age 1.

- Teach the parents to administer iron medication between meals and with citrus juice to maximize absorption. Advise them to give liquid medication through a straw or dropper, placing the medicine in the back of the child's mouth to avoid tooth staining.
- Ask the parents to describe the color of the child's stool, explaining that the stool of a child taking supplemental iron typically is dark green or black.
- Tell the parents that iron is toxic in high doses and must be locked away from the child to prevent accidental overdose. Advise them that if an overdose occurs, they should call the primary care practitioner or poison control center immediately.
- Enlist the assistance of a dietitian to work with the family if the diet is difficult to correct.
- Monitor the child's hemoglobin level and weight at monthly follow-up visits until both fall within normal ranges.

Leukemia

Progressive cancer of the blood-forming organs in which white blood cells (WBCs) and their precursors proliferate and develop abnormally in the blood and bone marrow.

NURSING DIAGNOSIS

Anxiety (parental) related to lack of knowledge about the child's condition and prognosis

DESIRED PATIENT OUTCOME

The parents will display increased knowledge and reduced anxiety about the child's condition

Outcome measurement criteria

- ☐ Verbalization by the parents of a basic understanding of leukemia and the need for treatment
- ☐ Description by the parents of what will occur during treatment
- ☐ Verbalization by the parents of the expected outcomes of treatment
- ☐ Expression by the parents of feelings about the diagnosis of cancer
- ☐ Verbalization by the parents of decreased anxiety about the child's condition
- ☐ Participation of the parents in the child's care
- ☐ Use by the parents of support from various sources

Key interventions

- Reinforce the primary care practitioner's explanation of leukemia and the need for treatment.

- Provide further information as questions arise. Also explain possible complications.
- Review the child's chemotherapy protocol and reinforce the primary care practitioner's explanation of chemotherapy and probable adverse effects.
- Encourage the family to minimize the child's trauma from chemotherapy's adverse effects by developing a routine to follow immediately after chemotherapy sessions, planning activities during expected periods of low WBC counts to minimize exposure to infection, applying ice to the child's head immediately after chemotherapy to decrease hair loss, obtaining a wig or cap for the child, and explaining the usual adverse effects to the child's siblings and friends.
- Reinforce the primary care practitioner's expectations about the outcome of treatment, encouraging questions and clarifying information.
- Encourage family members to express feelings and fears about the child's condition.
- Allow the child to play out fears using therapeutic play.
- Encourage the family to participate in the child's care.
- Encourage the parents to seek support from other family members and support groups.
- Arrange for the parents to meet with other families who have similar experiences.

NURSING DIAGNOSIS

Altered protection related to the body's decreased defenses

DESIRED PATIENT OUTCOME

The child will display no signs or symptoms of infection

Outcome measurement criteria

- ☐ Oral or tympanic temperature at or below 99° F (37.2° C); axillary temperature at or below 98° F (36.7° C)
- ☐ Clear breath sounds
- ☐ Age-appropriate pulse and respiratory rates
- ☐ Intact skin and mucous membranes
- ☐ Demonstration by the parents and child (if age-appropriate) of correct handwashing technique
- ☐ WBC count within normal limits
- ☐ Negative results on culture of specimens

Key interventions

- Monitor the child's temperature every 4 hours.
- Administer an antipyretic as prescribed if the oral or tympanic temperature exceeds 101° F (38.3° C) or if the axillary temperature exceeds 100° F (37.8° C). Take the temperature 1 hour after administration to determine the child's response to the antipyretic.
- Use nonpharmacologic methods to reduce fever, such as cool room temperature, fewer clothes and bedcovers, and tepid sponge baths.
- Monitor breath and heart sounds and pulse and respiratory rates.
- Assess for signs of infection in the skin (such as areas of skin breakdown) and mucous membranes (such as oral lesions).
- Teach the parents and child to wash their hands frequently, using proper handwashing technique.
- Use aseptic technique during procedures.
- Monitor the WBC count and the results of specimen cultures.
- Isolate the child if the WBC count makes the child vulnerable to infections from others.

- Administer antibiotics and antifungals as prescribed.

NURSING DIAGNOSIS

Altered protection related to the response to chemotherapy

DESIRED PATIENT OUTCOME

The child will experience no chemotherapy-induced bleeding episodes

Outcome measurement criteria

☐ Absence of skin or mouth lesions that indicate bleeding

☐ Absence of other signs of bleeding

☐ Age-appropriate vital signs

☐ Laboratory test results within normal ranges

Key interventions

- Inspect the patient every 4 hours for signs of bleeding; check secretions and stool for occult blood.
- Administer platelets or other blood components as prescribed. Monitor reactions to blood products. Do not administer drugs, such as aspirin, that interfere with platelet activity.
- Handle the child gently. Avoid invasive procedures during bleeding episodes. Protect the child from potential injuries from falls, sharp objects, and other hazards.
- Monitor the child's vital signs every 4 hours.
- Monitor the child's hemoglobin level, hematocrit, prothrombin time, and partial thromboplastin time.

NURSING DIAGNOSIS

Altered nutrition: less than body requirements, related to the effects of chemotherapy

DESIRED PATIENT OUTCOME

The child will consume sufficient food and fluids to meet the body's needs

Outcome measurement criteria

- ☐ Age-appropriate food and fluid intake
- ☐ Relatively balanced intake and output
- ☐ Intact mucous membranes
- ☐ Age-appropriate weight

Key interventions

- Consult with the dietitian on ways to promote food intake during therapy.
- Develop an extensive list of the child's favorite foods.
- Provide balanced meals that include the child's favorite foods, high-calorie foods, and high-protein foods.
- Encourage the child to eat with other children or with parents and to eat frequent, small meals.
- Administer I.V. fluids as prescribed during hospitalization. Help the parents obtain I.V. nursing services at home, and teach them how to monitor I.V. fluids. Encourage the child to drink six to eight glasses of fluids daily when at home, if the child can retain fluids.
- Record fluid intake and output.
- Monitor urine color, clarity, and amount as well as frequency of urination; monitor stool color and consistency as well as frequency of bowel movements.
- Brush the child's teeth, using a soft toothbrush. Encourage the child to brush, if old enough and physically able.
- Assess mucous membranes. Provide medication to soothe and heal mouth lesions. If mucous membranes are irritated, provide soft and nonspicy foods.
- Weigh the hospitalized child daily; otherwise, weekly.

Shock

Syndrome characterized by hypotension, poor peripheral circulation, inadequate organ perfusion, impaired cellular nutrition, and metabolic imbalance. In children, hypovolemia is the usual cause of shock; less common causes include sepsis, pump failure, and anaphylaxis.

NURSING DIAGNOSIS

Fluid volume deficit related to blood loss

DESIRED PATIENT OUTCOME

The child will display adequate fluid volume

Outcome measurement criteria

☐ Vital signs within age-appropriate ranges

☐ Normal cardiac rhythm

☐ Strong and equal peripheral pulses

☐ Warm arms and legs

☐ Capillary refill time of less than 2 seconds

☐ Age-appropriate fluid intake and output

☐ Urine output of at least 1 ml/kg/hour

☐ Urine specific gravity within age-appropriate range

☐ Age-appropriate arterial blood gas (ABG) levels

☐ Electrolyte levels within normal ranges

☐ Moist mucous membranes and elastic skin turgor

Key interventions

- Assess the child's vital signs for signs of decreased blood volume. Using a monitor, assess the cardiac rhythm for irregularities.

- Assess the peripheral pulses, which should be strong and equal.
- Assess the skin temperature of the arms and legs.
- Assess the capillary refill time in the nails.
- Administer fluid boluses and vasoactive medications as prescribed, carefully noting the child's response to medications.
- Ensure that the prescribed amount of I.V. fluid is infused on time; monitor the I.V. infusion site and fluids.
- Strictly monitor fluid intake and output. Check urine specific gravity and urine output every hour. Output should be at least 1 ml/kg/hour.
- Monitor ABGs and serum levels of electrolytes, especially potassium.
- Assess the child's mucous membranes and skin turgor.

NURSING DIAGNOSIS

High risk for altered body temperature related to the effects of systemic infection

DESIRED PATIENT OUTCOME

The child will maintain a normal body temperature

Outcome measurement criteria

☐ Oral or tympanic temperature of 98° to 99° F (36.6° to 37.2° C); axillary temperature of 97° to 98° F (36.1° to 36.6° C)

☐ Negative results on culture tests of specimens

☐ Age-appropriate white blood cell (WBC) count

☐ Absence of seizures

Key interventions

- Monitor the temperature every hour while the child is critically ill and then every 4 hours.
- Administer a nonaspirin antipyretic as prescribed if the temperature reaches or exceeds 101° F (38.3° C).
- Notify the primary care practitioner if the fever does not respond to medication or if the temperature falls below normal.
- Place the child on a cooling mattress, if necessary.
- Remove some of the child's clothing, but be careful not to chill the child.
- Keep the room temperature comfortably cool.
- Follow appropriate isolation procedures to prevent the spread of infection.
- Obtain specimens from the child for culture tests as ordered. Monitor culture test results and report them to the primary care practitioner.
- Obtain blood specimens to monitor the WBC count.
- Inquire about allergies to antibiotics.
- Administer I.V. antibiotics at the prescribed rate. Monitor the I.V. site for signs of infection and infiltration. Also monitor peak and trough antibiotic levels.
- Take seizure precautions, such as padding the sides of the bed, and monitor the child for seizures. If seizures occur, describe the type of activity, body parts involved, and duration of seizures.

NURSING DIAGNOSIS

Ineffective breathing pattern related to the effects of shock

DESIRED PATIENT OUTCOME

The child will display an age-appropriate breathing pattern

Outcome measurement criteria

- ☐ Age-appropriate respiratory and pulse rates
- ☐ Clear breath sounds
- ☐ Alert child
- ☐ Age-appropriate ABG and oxygen saturation levels
- ☐ Capillary refill time of less than 2 seconds

Key interventions

- Observe the child's respirations, particularly noting their rate, rhythm, depth, and symmetry as well as accessory muscle use.
- Auscultate the lungs to assess breath sounds.
- Position the child to promote effective respirations.
- Administer oxygen, as ordered.
- Monitor the child's apical pulse rate.
- Document the child's level of consciousness (LOC). Report decreasing LOC to the primary care practitioner.
- Monitor ABG and oxygen saturation (by pulse oximetry) levels. Report abnormal results to the primary care practitioner.
- Assess capillary refill time in the nails when monitoring vital signs, typically once every hour until the child is stable and then once every 4 hours.

NURSING DIAGNOSIS

High risk for injury (complications) related to ischemia

DESIRED PATIENT OUTCOME

The child will maintain sufficient blood flow to sustain cell life

Outcome measurement criteria

- ☐ Alert child
- ☐ Age-appropriate vital signs and body weight
- ☐ Absence of edema and ascites
- ☐ Balanced fluid intake and output
- ☐ Normal bowel sounds
- ☐ Absence of abdominal pain, nausea, and vomiting
- ☐ Absence of frank bleeding and occult blood in body excretions
- ☐ Age-appropriate urine specific gravity and serum creatinine, hemoglobin, and electrolyte levels

Key interventions

- Perform a neurologic assessment every hour. Report decreasing LOC to the primary care practitioner.
- Monitor the child's vital signs every hour. Notify the primary care practitioner of vital sign changes.
- Weigh the child at the same time every day, using the same scales and having the child wear the same amount of clothing.
- Assess for and document edema and ascites. If edema is detected, describe its location and grade.
- Strictly monitor the child's fluid intake and output.
- Help the child maintain the prescribed position in bed.
- Auscultate for bowel sounds every 4 hours. If they are absent, notify the primary care practitioner.
- Assess the child for nausea, vomiting, and abdominal pain, using the children's pain scale.
- Test vomitus and stool for occult blood.
- Check urine specific gravity every 4 hours.
- Monitor the child's serum creatinine, hemoglobin, and serum electrolyte levels, as ordered.

Sickle cell anemia

Inherited defect of hemoglobin synthesis in which sickle-shaped red blood cells (RBCs) replace normal, round RBCs; the sickling occurs when blood oxygenation or pH is decreased or dehydration occurs.

NURSING DIAGNOSIS

Anxiety (parental) related to lack of knowledge about the child's condition and care

DESIRED PATIENT OUTCOME

The parents will display increased knowledge and reduced anxiety about the child's condition and care

Outcome measurement criteria

- ☐ Demonstration by the parents of a basic knowledge about sickle cell anemia and related care
- ☐ Verbalization by the parents of feelings about the child's inheritance of a serious disease and about the presence of the disease in a parent, if applicable
- ☐ Statement by the parents that the outcome for the child depends on the quality of care and, to some extent, the family's involvement in care
- ☐ Identification by the parents of ways to prevent sickling episodes
- ☐ Verbalization by the parents of increased comfort with the child's condition

Key interventions

- Reinforce the primary care practitioner's explanation of the child's condition and the need to follow the prescribed treatment regimen, answering questions and clarifying information as needed.
- Encourage the parents to express feelings about the child's inheritance of a serious disease.
- Teach the parents how to prevent cell sickling by maintaining hydration. Instruct them to provide 100 to 125 ml/kg/day of fluids and calculate the number of glasses of fluids needed daily, provide favorite drinks, and prohibit strenuous activities. Advise them that the child is especially vulnerable to dehydration in the summer.
- Also advise the parents to watch for signs of impending dehydration, such as dry mouth, weight loss, thirst, and irritability, and to rehydrate the child if these signs occur.
- Teach the parents how to prevent cell sickling by avoiding infections. Instruct them to provide immunizations, including pneumococcal vaccine and *Haemophilus* b conjugate vaccine; protect the child from obvious sources of infection, such as large crowds and ill people; and watch for signs of infection, such as fever, cough, and sore throat.
- Teach the parents additional ways to prevent cell sickling. Suggest that they avoid exposing the child to high altitudes and nonpressurized planes; help the child identify and avoid stress and use stress-reduction techniques; encourage a balanced, high-calorie, high-protein diet and sufficient rest; and arrange for frequent checkups by the primary care practitioner.
- Instruct the parents to have the child wear a medical identification bracelet.
- Refer the family for genetic counseling.

NURSING DIAGNOSIS

Pain related to the effects of cell sickling

DESIRED PATIENT OUTCOME

The child will display increased comfort

Outcome measurement criteria

- □ Verbalization by the child (if age-appropriate) of increased comfort
- □ Demonstration by the child of increased comfort through smiling, talking, and playing
- □ Demonstration of increased comfort on the age-appropriate children's pain scale
- □ Expression by the parents and child (if age-appropriate) of feelings about painful episodes

Key interventions

- Ask the parents to identify measures that effectively relieve the child's pain.
- Administer oxygen and blood transfusions as prescribed. Provide adequate hydration by the I.V. and oral routes. Encourage bed rest to conserve oxygen and decrease pain.
- Assess the level of pain, using the age-appropriate children's pain scale.
- Administer nonaspirin analgesics on a schedule as prescribed. Recognize that patient-controlled analgesia, biofeedback, and imagery may be effective for older children.
- Determine the effectiveness of analgesics and nonpharmacologic pain-relief measures, using the age-appropriate children's pain scale.
- Apply a heating pad to the painful area if helpful.

- Provide nonstressful diversionary activities.
- Encourage the parents and child to express feelings about painful episodes.
- Provide opportunities for the younger child to play out painful experiences using dolls or hand puppets; urge the older child to talk about them.

NURSING DIAGNOSIS

High risk for fluid volume deficit related to the effects of infection

DESIRED PATIENT OUTCOME

The child will maintain adequate fluid volume

Outcome measurement criteria

☐ Relatively balanced fluid intake and urine output

☐ Moist mucous membranes and elastic skin turgor

☐ Urine specific gravity within normal range

☐ Age-appropriate serum electrolyte values

☐ Return to pre-crisis weight

Key interventions

- Keep a strict fluid intake and output record. Promote fluid intake by offering favorite drinks.
- Monitor I.V. fluid intake, and check the I.V. site for infiltration and erythema.
- Check the child's mucous membranes and skin turgor once every shift.
- Check urine specific gravity at every voiding.
- Monitor serum electrolyte values.
- Weigh the child daily.

Clubfoot, congenital

Foot deformity, present at birth, that usually involves foot inversion and adduction with plantar flexion (talipes equinovarus).

NURSING DIAGNOSIS

High risk for impaired skin integrity related to the effects of wearing a cast or Denis Browne splint

DESIRED PATIENT OUTCOME

The child will maintain intact skin on the legs and feet

Outcome measurement criteria

- ☐ Absence of skin lesions
- ☐ Absence of reddened skin
- ☐ Properly fitted cast or splint
- ☐ Adequate, balanced dietary intake
- ☐ Verbalization by the parents of the importance of maintaining skin integrity
- ☐ Identification by the parents of symptoms to report immediately to the primary care practitioner
- ☐ Demonstration by the parents of proper inspection of the cast and surrounding skin
- ☐ Attendance at follow-up appointments

Key interventions

- Teach the parents to inspect the cast edges for rough areas and to place tape over such areas.

- Advise the parents to notify the primary care practitioner if the cast seems to be getting tight. Inform them that casts usually are changed frequently as the child grows.
- Explain the risks of skin breakdown and instruct the parents to inspect the skin around the cast edges for signs of breakdown or irritation, to place padding between the cast and skin, and to apply the prescribed skin ointment. Advise them to note odor from the cast, which may signal infection, and to report it to the primary care practitioner.
- Tell the parents to check for pulses in the feet and circulation in the toes and to notify the primary care practitioner immediately if the toes are cold, discolored, or swollen.
- Advise the parents of the child with a Denis Browne splint to inspect the feet for skin breakdown or irritation; to apply prescribed ointment to the skin; to place a small, flat dressing on an open lesion to prevent contamination; and to remove the dressing to let the lesion dry when the splint is off.
- Provide the parents with nutritional information that is appropriate for the child's age, emphasizing the need for adequate fluids and nutrients to promote healthy skin, healing, and elimination.
- Stress the need to keep follow-up appointments.

NURSING DIAGNOSIS

High risk for altered growth and development related to immobilization

DESIRED PATIENT OUTCOME

The child will achieve optimum growth and development

Outcome measurement criteria

- ☐ Verbalization by the parents of age-appropriate growth and development norms for the child
- ☐ Use of appropriate support services
- ☐ Description by the parents of activities that promote growth and development
- ☐ Demonstration by the child of age-appropriate tasks and skills
- ☐ Age-appropriate weight and length

Key interventions

- Teach the parents the age-appropriate developmental milestones and growth norms.
- Urge the parents to use a physical therapist and other support services to help the child meet age-appropriate norms.
- Teach the parents age-appropriate activities that will promote the child's normal growth and development.
- Administer the Denver II Developmental Screening Test, noting any delays.
- Observe the child's behavior, and verify with the parents that the child is reaching milestones.
- Measure and plot the child's weight and length at follow-up visits, observing for age-appropriate growth.

Fracture

Interruption in bone continuity caused by trauma or disease.

NURSING DIAGNOSIS

Pain related to the effects of bone trauma or disease

DESIRED PATIENT OUTCOME

The child will report or demonstrate increased comfort

Outcome measurement criteria

☐ Verbalization by the parents and child (if age-appropriate) of feelings about painful experiences

☐ Demonstration by the child of increased comfort on the age-appropriate children's pain scale

☐ Choices by the child of measures that increase comfort

☐ Verbalization by the child (if age-appropriate) of increased comfort

☐ Demonstration by the child of increased comfort through smiling, talking, and playing, as age-appropriate

☐ Demonstration by the parents of how to handle the cast and inspect for signs of circulatory compromise

☐ Verbalization by the parents of appropriate home care measures

Key interventions

- Encourage the parents and child (if age-appropriate) to express feelings about painful experiences.
- Be truthful about painful treatments, indicating how much pain to expect and how long it will last.

- Use the age-appropriate children's pain scale to assess pain before and 30 minutes after administering pain medication.
- Administer the prescribed pain medication 30 minutes before cast application, if the child will be awake during the procedure.
- Provide privacy during cast application.
- Allow the parents to be present during cast application, if health care facility policy permits and the parents desire it.
- Encourage the child to hold still during cast application, assuring that the child may express pain by crying and yelling. Praise the child for holding still.
- Instruct the parents to avoid denting or damaging the cast; check toes or fingers for blueness, coldness, numbness, or swelling; and notify the primary care practitioner if any of these occurs.
- Teach the parents how to care for the child immediately after the injury. Advise them to administer the prescribed pain medication regularly, such as every 4 hours for the first 48 hours and then as needed; to assess for pain relief and notify the primary care practitioner if it is not adequate; to use pillows to elevate the limb above heart level if the child is lying down; to support the limb with a sling for an affected arm or a stool with pillows for an affected leg, if the child is sitting up; to place an ice bag over the fracture site during the first 48 hours; to distract the child in pain by reading aloud or providing music, television, or games; to let the child play out painful experiences; and to ask the child which pain-relief measures help the most.

NURSING DIAGNOSIS

High risk for impaired skin integrity related to lack of parental knowledge about required care

DESIRED PATIENT OUTCOME

The child will maintain intact skin

Outcome measurement criteria

- ☐ Verbalization by the parents of knowledge about fractures
- ☐ Description by the parents of the care needed to maintain skin integrity
- ☐ Identification by the parents of signs and symptoms to report immediately to the primary care practitioner
- ☐ Absence of skin lesions, redness, and signs of infection
- ☐ Properly fitted cast
- ☐ Demonstration by the parents of proper inspection of the cast and surrounding skin

Key interventions

- Teach the parents about the child's condition.
- Explain the purpose of the cast and its role in correcting the child's condition.
- Teach the parents to inspect the cast edges for rough areas and to place tape over these areas; inspect the skin around the cast edges for breakdown or irritation and—if found—keep the skin clean and dry, apply the prescribed ointment, and correct the irritation source; note and report odor from the cast, which may indicate infection; check feet or hands distal to the cast and immediately report coldness, discoloration, or swelling; check the cast for proper fit; plan to change the cast as the child grows; avoid placing sharp objects in the cast; prevent the child from getting sand or dirt inside the cast; provide toys that are too large for the child to put inside the cast; and use a large bib so food particles do not drop into the cast.
- Instruct the parents about the importance of adequate food and fluid intake in maintaining skin integrity.

Hip dysplasia, congenital

Hip defect, present at birth, in which the acetabulum is abnormally shallow, causing the head of the femur to fit incorrectly and possibly dislocate.

NURSING DIAGNOSIS

Altered peripheral tissue perfusion related to immobility

DESIRED PATIENT OUTCOME

The child will have adequate circulation to the legs

Outcome measurement criteria

- ☐ Adequate pedal pulses
- ☐ Toenail capillary refill time of less than 2 seconds
- ☐ Warm skin with normal color on feet and toes
- ☐ Absence of edema in feet
- ☐ Absence of pain on foot or leg movement

Key interventions

- Maintain correct positioning for a child in Bryant's traction by using a jacket restraint. This prevents the child from turning from side to side and placing uneven traction on the legs.
- Check that traction ropes pull evenly and weights hang freely.
- Rewrap the child's legs as prescribed by the primary care practitioner, carefully cleaning, drying, and examining the skin under the wraps. Do not apply lotion or oil. Document circulation assessments 30 minutes after rewrapping the legs.

- Check foot and leg circulation by palpating pedal pulses, checking capillary refill time in the toenails, and assessing skin color and temperature. Observe the feet for edema. Perform passive range-of-motion exercises on the feet, noting leg or foot pain with movement. Document assessments every 2 hours. Notify the primary care practitioner of pain or decreased circulation.

NURSING DIAGNOSIS

High risk for impaired skin integrity related to the parents' lack of knowledge about the child's disorder

DESIRED PATIENT OUTCOME

The child will maintain intact skin

Outcome measurement criteria

☐ Verbalization by the parents of knowledge of the child's disorder

☐ Identification by the parents of care needed to maintain skin integrity

☐ Verbalization by the parents of signs and symptoms to report immediately to the primary care practitioner

☐ Demonstration by the parents of appropriate cast-care techniques

☐ Absence of skin lesions, redness, and signs of infection

☐ Properly fitted harness or cast

☐ Age-appropriate food and fluid intake

☐ Attendance at follow-up appointments

Key interventions

- Teach the parents about the disorder, including how long the child will wear a Pavlik or other harness or body cast.

- Explain to the parents the purpose of the harness or cast and its role in correcting the child's hip defect.
- Teach the parents of a child with a harness to check it for proper fit, to follow the instructions for use, and to inspect the skin for redness or irritation and, if present, to keep the skin clean and dry and apply the prescribed ointment. Tell the parents to apply padding under the shoulder straps if the skin becomes irritated.
- Teach the parents of a child with a cast to inspect its edges for rough areas and to place tape over these areas; inspect the skin around the cast edges for signs of breakdown or irritation and—if present—to keep the skin clean and dry, apply the prescribed ointment, and correct the source of the irritation; note and report odor from the cast; check for pulses in the feet and circulation in the toes and immediately report cold, discolored, or swollen feet; check the cast for proper fit (a finger should fit between the top of the cast and the child's abdomen); plan to change the cast as the child grows; use a large bib during feeding so food particles do not drop into the cast; prevent the child from getting sand or dirt inside the cast; and provide toys that are too large for the child to put inside the cast. Advise the parents to protect the cast around the perineal area by tucking plastic wrap inside the cast and folding it over the outside edges to cover the cast, replacing the wrapping as needed, and using extra-absorbent diapers with elastic leg openings and tucking the diaper between the cast and the skin.
- Explain the importance of nutrition in maintaining skin integrity and other body functions. Advise the parents to provide a diet high in protein, calories, and calcium; to include high-fiber foods (if age-appropriate); and to provide age-appropriate quantities of fluids.
- Emphasize the need for follow-up appointments.

NURSING DIAGNOSIS

High risk for altered growth and development related to the effects of wearing a cast or other corrective device

DESIRED PATIENT OUTCOME

The child will attain normal growth and developmental milestones

Outcome measurement criteria

- ☐ Verbalization by the parents of age-appropriate growth and development norms for the child
- ☐ Use of appropriate support services
- ☐ Identification by the parents of activities that promote growth and development
- ☐ Demonstration by the child of age-appropriate skills
- ☐ Age-appropriate weight and length

Key interventions

- Teach the parents about age-appropriate developmental milestones and growth norms.
- Encourage the use of a physical therapist and other services to help meet age-appropriate milestones.
- Teach the parents age-appropriate play for the child to promote normal growth and development.
- Teach the parents to provide sensory stimulation for the child by putting toys in reach, moving the child to areas of activity in the house, or taking the child out in a cart.
- Administer the Denver II Developmental Screening Test, noting developmental delays.
- During follow-up visits, measure and plot the child's weight and length, observing for age-appropriate growth. Also, observe the child's behavior, and verify with the parents that the child is reaching milestones.

Osteomyelitis

Local or generalized infection of a bone.

NURSING DIAGNOSIS

Pain related to the effects of osteomyelitis

DESIRED PATIENT OUTCOME

The child will display increased comfort

Outcome measurement criteria

- ☐ Verbalization by the parents and child (if age-appropriate) of feelings about painful experiences
- ☐ Demonstration by the child of increased comfort on the age-appropriate children's pain scale
- ☐ Verbalization or demonstration by the child of increased comfort
- ☐ Choices by the child of measures that increase comfort

Key interventions

- Encourage the parents and child (if age-appropriate) to express feelings about painful experiences.
- Assess the intensity of pain and degree of pain relief using the age-appropriate children's pain scale.
- Administer prescribed medications to the child 30 minutes before a painful procedure or surgery.
- Be truthful about painful procedures, indicating how much pain to expect and how long it will last.
- Provide privacy during painful procedures.
- Allow the parents to be present during procedures if health care facility policy permits and the parents desire it.

- Encourage the child to hold still during procedures, assuring that the child may express pain by crying and yelling. Praise the child for holding still.
- Give the prescribed pain medication on schedule or by a patient-controlled analgesia pump, if the child is age 10 or older, during the first few days of therapy. Gradually switch to an oral pain medication as prescribed.
- Encourage the older child to ask for medication at the onset of pain, rather than waiting until pain is severe. For a younger child, ask the parents to request medication at the first sign of pain, such as irritability, whimpering, or restlessness.
- Handle the child gently, being especially careful with the affected body part.
- Provide distractions or use imagery in addition to medication for a child in pain.
- Let the child play out painful experiences using dolls or puppets; use a play therapist, if available.

NURSING DIAGNOSIS

High risk for altered growth and development related to the effects of long-term antibiotic treatment for osteomyelitis

DESIRED PATIENT OUTCOME

The child will display normal growth and development

Outcome measurement criteria

- ☐ Verbalization by the parents of age-appropriate growth and development norms
- ☐ Verbalization by the parents of the possible effects of hospitalization and outpatient therapy on growth and development

□ Age-appropriate growth, behavior, and development of social, communication, and intellectual skills by the child

Key interventions

- Teach the parents the age-appropriate growth and development norms.
- Teach the parents how treatment may affect the child's growth and development. Explain that noncompliance with the antibiotic regimen can cause relapse and rehospitalization, which reduces the child's opportunities for age-appropriate activities, such as gross motor play and school participation.
- Help the parents obtain home health care I.V. services for antibiotic administration to enable the child to attend school.
- Urge the parents to provide large amounts of fluids during antibiotic therapy to prevent urinary tract problems that could lead to rehospitalization.
- Encourage the parents to provide age-appropriate diversionary activities to promote development of social, communication, and intellectual skills.
- Evaluate the child's growth and social, communication, and intellectual skills during follow-up appointments; compare them with age-appropriate norms.

Rheumatoid arthritis, juvenile

Chronic autoimmune disease causing joint inflammation and pain.

NURSING DIAGNOSIS

Pain related to inflammation associated with juvenile rheumatoid arthritis

DESIRED PATIENT OUTCOME

The child will display increased comfort

Outcome measurement criteria

- ☐ Verbalization or demonstration by the child of comfort or, at least, tolerable pain
- ☐ Documentation by the child of a progressive decrease in pain on the age-appropriate children's pain scale
- ☐ Use of physical therapy as needed
- ☐ Movement of joints with minimal discomfort
- ☐ Engagement in activities of daily living (ADLs) and play

Key interventions

- Assess the level of pain using the age-appropriate children's pain scale.
- Teach the parents about prescribed medications. Advise them to administer medications consistently (unless discontinued by the primary care practitioner) with meals, to report signs of toxicity immediately, and to have serum drug levels monitored.
- Refer the child to a physical therapist, if needed.
- Describe measures to decrease pain and stiffness, such as warm baths and heat application on joints.

- Discuss joint splint use if joint movement is painful.
- Teach the child that maintaining one position for a prolonged period will increase pain and stiffness and that overusing joints will increase pain.
- Encourage the child to engage in self-care activities, including range-of-motion (ROM) exercises.
- Provide opportunities for play and exercise that avoid prolonged or strenuous activity.
- Encourage the parents to inform the child's teacher of the child's condition.

NURSING DIAGNOSIS

High risk for activity intolerance related to pain and fatigue secondary to juvenile rheumatoid arthritis

DESIRED PATIENT OUTCOME

The child will perform ADLs without undue fatigue

Outcome measurement criteria

- ☐ Verbalization by the child of decreased fatigue
- ☐ Verbalization by the parents that the child is more active
- ☐ Participation by the child in ADLs and play
- ☐ Age-appropriate vital signs during ADLs and play
- ☐ Adequate caloric and nutritional intake
- ☐ Normal hemoglobin and hematocrit levels

Key interventions

- Help the parents and child develop a plan that balances activity and rest and avoids strenuous or prolonged exercise. Teach the child to rest when pain or fatigue occurs.
- Assess the child's fatigue using a scale.

- Note how long the child is active before voluntarily resting.
- Note vital signs before and during activity; compare them with resting vital signs.
- Ask how long the child sleeps and compare this with age-appropriate norms.
- Assess the child's ability to play at the age-appropriate level before becoming fatigued.
- Evaluate the child's ability to perform age-appropriate self-care activities before becoming fatigued.
- Assess the child's food and fluid intake. Teach the parents and child (if age-appropriate) the importance of a well-balanced diet and adequate fluids.
- Monitor the child's hemoglobin and hematocrit levels.

NURSING DIAGNOSIS

High risk for altered health maintenance related to insufficient knowledge about home care

DESIRED PATIENT OUTCOME

The parents and child (if age-appropriate) will successfully manage the child's home care

Outcome measurement criteria

- ☐ Verbalization by the parents and child (if age-appropriate) of an understanding of the child's care
- ☐ Verbalization by the parents and child (if age-appropriate) of a mutual desire to cooperate in care
- ☐ Use by the parents and child (if age-appropriate) of support systems

Key interventions

- Discuss with the parents and child (if age-appropriate) the possible physical and psychological effects of juvenile rheumatoid arthritis.
- Teach the parents and child (if age-appropriate) about ROM and muscle-strengthening exercises; play activities, such as swimming and recreational dancing, that do not overtax the child's energy or joints; and stress-reduction techniques.
- Teach the parents and child (if age-appropriate) that the child should take aspirin with meals and should be monitored for adverse effects, including hearing problems or stomach upset. Stress the need for continued monitoring of the child's medications, symptoms, and laboratory values.
- Encourage the parents and child (if age-appropriate) to discuss feelings about the effects of the disease on their lives.
- Urge the family to use support systems, such as a physical therapist, other health care team members, patients and families coping with the same condition, the school nurse, and local and national Arthritis Foundations.

Scoliosis

Lateral curvature of the spine.

NURSING DIAGNOSIS

Anxiety related to lack of knowledge about scoliosis and its outcome

DESIRED PATIENT OUTCOME

The parents and child will demonstrate increased knowledge and reduced anxiety about scoliosis and its outcome

Outcome measurement criteria

- ☐ Verbalization by the parents and child of knowledge about scoliosis
- ☐ Discussion by the parents and child of concerns about scoliosis
- ☐ Description by the parents and child of treatments and anticipated outcomes
- ☐ Description by the parents and child of what to expect after treatments
- ☐ Verbalization by the parents and child of decreased anxiety

Key interventions

- Inform the family about scoliosis and its treatments and outcomes.
- Encourage the family to ask questions and discuss concerns about scoliosis and its treatments; correct inaccurate information.

- Tell the parents and child that if a brace is prescribed, it must be worn 23 of every 24 hours until bone growth stops, and then must be worn at night for about 2 more years or until the bones mature.
- Orient the parents and child to the waiting room and special care unit to which the child will return if surgery must be performed. Introduce the family to the staff members who will care for the child.
- Inform the parents and child about preoperative tests and use of the children's pain scale. Teach deep-breathing exercises.
- Explain to the parents that the child will receive preoperative medication to promote relaxation and will be taken to surgery on a stretcher.
- Explain to the parents that the child will be in a recovery area for 1½ to 2 hours after surgery; that health care facility policy will determine whether the parents can stay with the child in the recovery area; that vital signs, blood pressure, and the incision dressing will be checked every 15 minutes; and that the child will have an I.V. and catheter in place upon awakening.
- Explain that the child will receive pain medication after surgery and will receive fluids and food as soon as the child can tolerate them.

NURSING DIAGNOSIS

Pain related to the effects of surgery for scoliosis

DESIRED PATIENT OUTCOME

The child will display increased comfort

Outcome measurement criteria

□ Verbalization by the parents and child of feelings about painful experiences

- ☐ Demonstration by the child of increased comfort on the children's pain scale
- ☐ Choices by the child of measures that increase comfort
- ☐ Verbalization or demonstration by the child of increased comfort

Key interventions

- Encourage the parents and child to express feelings about painful experiences.
- Ask the parents about the child's usual reaction to pain and about effective pain-relief measures.
- Administer prescribed analgesics regularly during the immediate postoperative period using the patient-controlled analgesia method. Determine the effects of analgesia on pain by using the children's pain scale.
- Involve the parents in pain-relief measures, such as distraction games, imagery, music, and relaxation techniques; encourage them to anticipate pain and offer relief measures before pain becomes severe; encourage the child (if age-appropriate) to tell the parents when pain starts.
- Help the child determine which pain-relief measures decrease pain.
- Note the child's level of interaction with the parents, staff, and environment, and document the child's apparent comfort.

NURSING DIAGNOSIS

High risk for altered health maintenance related to concerns secondary to adolescence

DESIRED PATIENT OUTCOME

The parents and child will successfully manage home care

Outcome measurement criteria

- ☐ Verbalization by the parents and child of knowledge and feelings about the child's condition
- ☐ Description by the parents and child of required home care
- ☐ Identification by the parents and child of appropriate exercise and activities
- ☐ Attendance at appointments with tne primary care practitioner
- ☐ Use by the parents and child of a physical therapist and appropriate support groups
- ☐ Absence of hospitalizations due to lack of adequate care
- ☐ Verbalization by the parents and child of satisfaction with home care

Key interventions

- Teach the parents and child about scoiiosis and its treatment before the child's discharge. Discuss the eventual benefits of treatment for scoliosis.
- Discuss the child's home care needs, explaining that a brace (if prescribed) must be worn for 23 of every 24 hours, that the parents must check the child's skin for signs of irritation, and that they must apply the prescribed ointment to the irritation site and place a pad over it for protection.
- Teach ways to increase comfort while wearing a brace, such as allowing the child to purchase clothes that fit easily over the brace; encouraging concentration on aspects of appearance that the child can control, such as hair and makeup; and encouraging the child to vent feelings about the brace.
- Instruct the parents of the child who has had surgery to check for increased pain at the incision site or down the leg, note drainage or odor, and notify the surgeon if

increased pain or drainage or odor occurs; to prohibit the child from bathing until the surgeon allows; and to take the temperature daily, notifying the surgeon if fever develops. Review the child's activity limitations and discuss when the child can return to school.

- Advise the parents to provide a firm mattress for the child's bed; consult a physical therapist about measures that will promote comfort, especially when sleeping in a brace.
- Stress to the parents and child the need for the primary care practitioner to continually monitor the child's condition.
- Promote the parents' and child's use of support systems, such as the National Scoliosis Foundation. Arrange for the child to meet with others being treated for scoliosis. Encourage the adolescent to express feelings about the effects of the disease on his or her life, including activity and clothing restrictions.

Cerebral palsy

A permanent, nonprogressive motor disorder caused by damage to the central nervous system and characterized by impairment of voluntary movement.

NURSING DIAGNOSIS

Grieving (parental) related to loss of the child's health

DESIRED PATIENT OUTCOME

The parents will cope effectively with grief associated with loss of the child's health

Outcome measurement criteria

- □ Verbalization by the parents of an understanding of grief
- □ Expressions of grief by the parents
- □ Verbalization by the parents of support for each other
- □ Expressions of support by the extended family
- □ Verbalization by the parents of a plan to manage the initial phases of their adjustment to the situation

Key interventions

- Assess the family's experiences with grief and loss, and learn how grief was resolved. Identify the family's strengths as a unit and as individuals.
- Explain that grief is normal; clarify misconceptions.
- Encourage the parents to express feelings about cerebral palsy and loss of their child's health.

- Encourage the parents to be truthful with other family members.
- Prepare the parents for possible responses of people outside the immediate family to the child's cerebral palsy.
- Encourage family members to demonstrate love and support for each other.
- Discuss ways to manage the immediate situation, including caring for the family's other children, making arrangements with employers, and planning for financial considerations.

NURSING DIAGNOSIS

Anxiety (parental) related to lack of knowledge about cerebral palsy and required care

DESIRED PATIENT OUTCOME

The parents will display increased knowledge and reduced anxiety about cerebral palsy

Outcome measurement criteria

- ☐ Verbalization of basic knowledge about cerebral palsy
- ☐ Description of normal growth and development that the child should demonstrate
- ☐ Discussion of concerns about the child's disorder
- ☐ Verbalization of the need for assistance to maximize the child's potential
- ☐ Verbalization of decreased anxiety about the child's disorder and care

Key interventions

- Discuss cerebral palsy and encourage the parents to discuss their concerns about its effect on the child. Invite family members to ask questions.

- Discuss normal growth and development and the potential variations from norms that the child may experience.
- Urge the parents to commit to maximizing the child's potential while maintaining realistic expectations.
- Encourage the family to identify care tasks that are anxiety-producing. Then provide instructions about those tasks and work with the family until they feel comfortable doing them.
- Involve the parents in community and facility support groups.

NURSING DIAGNOSIS

High risk for altered nutrition: less than body requirements, related to difficulty with sucking and swallowing

DESIRED PATIENT OUTCOME

The child will maintain age-appropriate dietary intake

Outcome measurement criteria

- ☐ Verbalization by the parents of the importance of adequate dietary intake
- ☐ Age-appropriate weight
- ☐ Age-appropriate dietary intake
- ☐ Use of appropriate support services
- ☐ Laboratory serum values indicating adequate nutrition

Key interventions

- Discuss with the parents the importance of the child's dietary intake, answering questions about nutrition and clarifying the signs and effects of malnutrition.

- Weigh the child weekly at the same time, using the same scale, and with the child wearing the same amount of clothing.
- Consult an occupational therapist. Teach the family to use adaptive feeding and drinking devices, if appropriate, and to feed the child slowly, using manual jaw control.
- Consult a dietitian and collaborate on a plan for meeting the child's nutritional needs.
- Teach the parents to offer frequent, small meals and to provide a high-carbohydrate diet using sample menus they have prepared with the dietitian and nurse.
- Have the parents record food intake, administer the prescribed vitamins and minerals, and obtain regular evaluations of all intake by the nurse or dietitian.
- Schedule physical therapy and exercise sessions no sooner than 2 hours after meals.
- Check laboratory serum values on follow-up visits.

NURSING DIAGNOSIS

High risk for impaired home maintenance management related to the complexity of care

DESIRED PATIENT OUTCOME

The parents will successfully manage the home care regimen

Outcome measurement criteria

- ☐ Verbalization by the parents of the need for consistent, long-term care
- ☐ Verbalization by the parents of concerns about home care
- ☐ Explanation by the parents of the child's condition and required home care

- ☐ Demonstration by the parents of appropriate feeding methods
- ☐ Age-appropriate weight
- ☐ Verbalization by the parents of the need to monitor the child's elimination patterns
- ☐ Demonstration by the parents of arm and leg exercises
- ☐ Verbalization by the parents of the need for seizure medication
- ☐ Verbalization by the parents of realistic goals for the child
- ☐ Use by the family of appropriate community resources
- ☐ Absence of hospitalizations due to inadequate care

Key interventions

- Discuss the need for long-term care for the child. Encourage the parents to discuss concerns about home care.
- Teach the parents about nutrition-related home care. Advise them to follow the occupational therapist's suggestions for feeding with assistive devices and manual jaw control; slowly feed mashed or soft foods to the child who has difficulty chewing or swallowing, place foods farther back in the mouth if the child has difficulty swallowing or has tongue thrusting, determine the child's food preferences and use as many as possible, give high-carbohydrate foods, administer prescribed vitamins and minerals, and weigh the child weekly at same time, using the same scale, and with the child wearing same amount of clothing.
- Teach the parents how to meet the child's elimination needs at home. Advise them to develop a urine and bowel schedule to avoid incontinence and ensure adequate elimination, note the color and clarity of the urine and color and consistency of stools, and alert the primary care practitioner if urine or stools appear abnor-

mal; to catheterize the child, if needed; and to use suppositories or digital stimulation to stimulate bowel movement.

- Advise the parents to follow the exercise program developed by the physical therapist, to keep appointments for physical therapy, and to provide opportunities for locomotion using mobilizing devices, such as braces or wheeled devices.
- Advise the parents of the child with seizures to give seizure medication regularly, to protect the child from self-injury during seizures by moving the child away from objects that might cause injury and turning the child's head to the side to prevent aspiration, and to keep appointments for assessing medication blood levels.
- Teach the parents to enhance the child's educational opportunities by developing the child's speech and communication skills through using the plan developed by the speech therapist; creating a communication system for the child, if necessary, such as one using eye blinks or computers; having the child's intellectual capacity evaluated; setting realistic goals for the child; and praising and encouraging the child.
- Refer the parents and child to family and community resources. Suggest ways in which the extended family can help, such as baby-sitting and providing respite care or transportation. Contact appropriate community agencies and facilitate their use by the family. Encourage the use of early intervention programs, and make the family aware of financial assistance programs.

NURSING DIAGNOSIS

High risk for body image disturbance related to the effects of cerebral palsy

DESIRED PATIENT OUTCOME

The child will display a positive body image

Outcome measurement criteria

- ☐ Communication of positive statements about abilities
- ☐ Communication of positive aspects of appearance
- ☐ Participation in self-care and social activities

Key interventions

- Encourage the child to express feelings to the family about his or her abilities and appearance.
- Identify the child's strengths and abilities and discuss ways to enhance them, including the family in the discussion if the child desires.
- Have the child list positive aspects of his or her appearance. Encourage the child to ask a parent, sibling, or friend for a different perspective.
- Advise the parents to encourage the child to perform as much self-care as possible and to actively participate in grooming, choosing clothes, and styling hair.
- Discuss how the child feels about his or her current appearance and what will enhance it.
- Encourage the parents and child to participate in social and other activities outside the home, such as shopping and attending church or sports events.
- Encourage the parents' and child's participation in support groups and camps for children with special needs.

Head trauma

Wound or injury to the brain or tissues inside the head.

NURSING DIAGNOSIS

High risk for injury related to the effects of head trauma

DESIRED PATIENT OUTCOME

The child will have no injuries due to the effects of head trauma

Outcome measurement criteria

- ☐ Normal neurologic signs
- ☐ Age-appropriate intracranial pressure (ICP)
- ☐ Age-appropriate urine output and urine specific gravity
- ☐ Patent airway
- ☐ Normal vital signs
- ☐ Arterial blood gas (ABG), serum pH, and serum electrolyte values within normal ranges
- ☐ Intact skin
- ☐ Normal gag, swallow, and blink reflexes

Key interventions

- Record neurologic checks and neurologic effects every hour. Notify the primary care practitioner of deterioration.
- Monitor ICP and calculate cerebral perfusion pressure. Notify the primary care practitioner of an abrupt increase or serial increases in ICP.

- Elevate the head of the bed to 30 degrees, maintain the child's head in the midline position, and minimize stimuli, such as noise, light, touch, and pain.
- Administer prescribed medications to help keep ICP within the normal range.
- Administer I.V. solutions exactly as prescribed and maintain strict fluid intake and output records. Notify the primary care practitioner if output is less than 1 ml/kg/hour.
- Provide indwelling urinary catheter care, check urine specific gravity every 2 hours, and monitor serum electrolyte and pH levels.
- Assess for the gag and swallowing reflexes.
- Maintain a patent airway, suctioning only if essential and hyperventilating the child before and after suctioning. Record the character of secretions.
- Auscultate the chest every 2 hours and monitor pulse and respiratory rates and blood pressure. Notify the primary care practitioner of abnormal findings.
- Monitor ABG values. Notify the primary care practitioner if abnormal values do not respond to interventions.
- Inspect the skin while providing other care. Also, coordinate care to minimize stimulation, gently perform range-of-motion (ROM) exercises and turn the patient if ICP is within the normal range, and use an egg-crate mattress cover.
- Monitor for the blink reflex. If the reflex is absent, keep the eyelids closed and instill prescribed eye drops.

NURSING DIAGNOSIS

High risk for altered health maintenance related to lack of knowledge about caring for the child with head trauma

DESIRED PATIENT OUTCOME

The parents will successfully manage the child's care

Outcome measurement criteria

- ☐ Verbalization by the parents of an understanding of the child's condition and prognosis
- ☐ Verbalization by the parents of the signs and symptoms to report to the primary care practitioner
- ☐ Description by the parents of required home care and its importance
- ☐ Demonstration by the parents of necessary home care skills
- ☐ Verbalization by the parents of comfort with managing home care
- ☐ Use by the family of support systems and groups

Key interventions

- Reinforce the primary care practitioner's discussion of the child's condition and prognosis, encouraging the parents to ask questions and clarifying information.
- Discuss realistic expectations for the child, and help the parents develop a care plan.
- Teach the parents the signs and symptoms to report immediately to the primary care practitioner: asymmetrical pupils, prolonged staring or unusual eye movements, breathing difficulty, anterior fontanel bulging in a child under age 18 months, change in or unusual behavior, excessive sleeping and difficulty being aroused, fever, redness or purulence around tube entry sites, lack of urination or bowel movements, loss of or change in bladder and bowel control, inadequate fluid or food intake, projectile vomiting, and unusual arm and leg weakness.

- Discuss home care, including bowel and urinary care, breathing treatments, exercise, activity, nutrition, skin care, and temperature monitoring.
- Demonstrate the skills needed to care for the child and have the parents return the demonstration of these skills: feeding, suctioning, taking the temperature, monitoring the ventilator and I.V. therapy, and administering catheter care, suppositories, breathing treatments, ROM exercises, and medications.
- Provide telephone numbers to call when questions about care arise.
- Help the family use community agencies for assistance with home care.
- Teach the parents how to manage seizures. (For details, see the "Seizures" entry in this section.)

Hydrocephalus

Accumulation of an abnormally large amount of cerebrospinal fluid in the cranium resulting from a structural anomaly, tumor, infection, or trauma.

NURSING DIAGNOSIS

High risk for injury related to the effects of hydrocephalus

DESIRED PATIENT OUTCOME

The child will sustain no injury to the head or neck

Outcome measurement criteria

- ☐ Verbalization by the parents of the need to support the child's head and of the child's inability to move the head
- ☐ Verbalization by the parents of appropriate positioning of the child's head
- ☐ Absence of injuries to the child's head or neck
- ☐ Verbalization by the parents of the need to give special care to the child's scalp
- ☐ Intact skin on the child's head

Key interventions

- Advise the parents to always support the child's head.
- Monitor the child's skin for redness or purulence at shunt incision sites and redness or lesions on the skin over the shunt tubing or on the scalp because of the weight of the head.
- Teach the parents to turn the child's head every 2 hours.
- Protect the child's head from pressure caused by hard objects, such as the bed frame or toys.

NURSING DIAGNOSIS

Anxiety (parental) related to lack of knowledge about hydrocephalus and related home care

DESIRED PATIENT OUTCOME

The parents will demonstrate reduced anxiety and will successfully manage home care

Outcome measurement criteria

- ☐ Verbalization of knowledge about hydrocephalus
- ☐ Description of required treatments and anticipated outcomes
- ☐ Expression of concerns
- ☐ Verbalization of decreased anxiety
- ☐ Verbalization of the care needed for the child
- ☐ Demonstration of the skills needed to care for the child
- ☐ Participation in the child's care
- ☐ Verbalization of the signs and symptoms to report immediately to the primary care practitioner
- ☐ Use of community support systems

Key interventions

- Reinforce the primary care practitioner's explanations about the child's condition, treatments, and prognosis. Clarify information as needed.
- Discuss with the parents their concerns about the child's disorder, care, and prognosis.
- Teach the parents about home care, including caring for the scalp; verifying shunt patency by pressing the valve as prescribed and noting if the valve fills with fluid; monitoring the temperature; checking for signs of increased intracranial pressure (ICP), such as a bulging fontanel or increased head size if the child is under age

18 months, projectile vomiting, difficulty being aroused, difficulty in speaking or swallowing, fever, unusual eye movements or staring, and uneven pupils; supporting the child's head; and monitoring the child during a seizure, noting its length and associated movements and protecting the child by turning the head to the side to drain saliva and removing objects that could cause injury.

- Demonstrate the necessary home care skills, such as pumping the shunt and taking the temperature. Have the parents return the demonstration.
- Teach the parents the signs and symptoms to report immediately to the primary care practitioner: fever, inadequate food or fluid intake, breathing difficulty, seizures, and signs of increased ICP.
- Provide telephone numbers to call when questions about care arise.
- Facilitate the parents' use of community support agencies.

NURSING DIAGNOSIS

High risk for caregiver role strain related to the demands of long-term care

DESIRED PATIENT OUTCOME

The parents will maintain physical and mental health

Outcome measurement criteria

□ Verbalization by the parents of positive attitudes toward the child and care responsibilities

□ Signs of physical and mental health of the parents

□ Willingness of the parents to use support services

□ Willingness of the parents to use respite care

□ Demonstration of support by other family members

Key interventions

- Encourage the parents to discuss feelings about care.
- Encourage the parents to have regular physical check-ups.
- Develop a plan for family members to share in care.
- Discuss the importance of having a respite from caregiving, such as an evening out or an occasional overnight trip.
- Encourage family members to provide mutual support, demonstrate caring attitudes, and acknowledge one another's contributions.
- Refer the parents to appropriate community support agencies and promote their use by the family.

Myelomeningocele

Developmental anomaly that allows the spinal cord and meninges to protrude through a defect in the vertebral column.

NURSING DIAGNOSIS

Anxiety (parental) related to lack of knowledge about the disorder

DESIRED PATIENT OUTCOME

The parents will display increased knowledge and reduced anxiety about the child's disorder

Outcome measurement criteria

- ☐ Verbalization by the parents and child (if age-appropriate) of knowledge about myelomeningocele
- ☐ Description by the parents of the necessary treatment and anticipated outcome
- ☐ Verbalization by the parents of concerns about the disorder
- ☐ Verbalization by the parents of decreased anxiety
- ☐ Participation by the parents in the child's care

Key interventions

- Reinforce the information given to the parents by the primary care practitioner about the child's disorder, treatments, and expected outcome. Encourage questions and clarify information.
- Urge the parents to discuss concerns about the disorder.
- Encourage the parents to participate in the child's care as much as possible.

- Refer the parents to appropriate support groups, if needed.

NURSING DIAGNOSIS

Grieving (parental) related to loss of the child's health

DESIRED PATIENT OUTCOME

The parents will cope effectively with grief related to the loss of the child's health

Outcome measurement criteria

- ☐ Expressions of grief by the parents
- ☐ Verbalization by the parents that reflects an understanding of grieving
- ☐ Verbalization by the parents of the effects of caregiving on the family's lifestyle
- ☐ Demonstration of mutual support by family members
- ☐ Verbalization by the parents of a plan to deal with the immediate details of caring for the child

Key interventions

- Assess the parents' experiences with grief and loss.
- Explain that grief is normal, describing each stage of grieving and clarifying misconceptions.
- Encourage the parents to discuss feelings about the loss of the child's health and the prognosis of chronic impairment.
- Identify the family's strengths as a unit and as individuals.
- Encourage the parents to be open and truthful with family members. Prepare them for the possible responses of others to the child's condition.

- Discuss ways for the parents to deal with the immediate details of caring for the child, such as providing adequate care for the child and siblings; making special arrangements with employers, as needed; making financial arrangements for the child's care; and modifying the home environment as needed.

NURSING DIAGNOSIS

High risk for infection related to the effects of a spinal defect

DESIRED PATIENT OUTCOME

The child will remain free from infection

Outcome measurement criteria

- ☐ Absence of fluid leakage from the sac
- ☐ Absence of signs of localized infection
- ☐ Tympanic temperature at or below 99° F (37.2° C)
- ☐ Negative results of sac fluid cultures
- ☐ Age-appropriate white blood cell (WBC) count

Key interventions

- Use sterile gloves when handling the infant and avoid pressure on the sac.
- Place the child on the abdomen on sterile sheets. Position the legs and feet appropriately and turn the head every 2 hours.
- Apply the prescribed solution or cream and a sterile dressing to the sac. Do not place diapers or covers over the sac, but protect the sac area from urine and feces.
- Immediately report fluid leakage from the sac.
- Observe the sac every 4 hours for redness or purulence.
- Monitor the tympanic temperature every 4 hours.

- Obtain a specimen of exudate or fluid around the sac area for culture as prescribed.
- Monitor the WBC count and report abnormal values.

NURSING DIAGNOSIS

Impaired physical mobility related to the effects of myelomeningocele

DESIRED PATIENT OUTCOME

The child will display as much mobility as possible

Outcome measurement criteria

- ☐ Verbalization by the parents of the need to maintain the child's mobility
- ☐ Demonstration by the parents of how to perform range-of-motion (ROM) exercises on the child's joints
- ☐ Demonstration by the parents of the appropriate use of assistive devices
- ☐ Keeping by the parents of appointments with the primary care practitioner and physical therapist

Key interventions

- Explain the need for continuous care to increase the child's mobility and prevent further limitations.
- Teach the parents to exercise the child's legs with strengthening and ROM exercises at morning and night; to align the child correctly while in a bed or chair; to develop a schedule for the child to change position; to teach the child to shift weight every 15 minutes while sitting; to monitor the skin over bony body areas and pressure points under braces; to contact the primary care practitioner if a reddened area develops; to apply assistive devices, such as braces, correctly; to assess the child for correct use of braces and crutches; and to urge

the child to be as independent as possible.

- Impress on the parents the need for continued physical therapy and medical monitoring.

NURSING DIAGNOSIS

High risk for caregiver role strain related to the complexity of long-term care

DESIRED PATIENT OUTCOME

The parents will maintain optimum physical and mental health

Outcome measurement criteria

- ☐ Verbalization by the parents of a positive attitude toward the child and care responsibilities
- ☐ Signs of physical health of the parents
- ☐ Willingness of the parents to use support services
- ☐ Willingness of the parents to participate in respite care
- ☐ Demonstration of support by other family members

Key interventions

- Encourage the parents to discuss feelings about care.
- Encourage the parents to have regular checkups.
- Develop a plan in which family members share in care.
- Discuss the importance of having a respite from caregiving, such as an evening out.
- Refer the parents to appropriate community support agencies and facilitate their use.
- Encourage family members to provide mutual support and acknowledge one another's contributions.
- Teach the parents how to cope with seizures. (For details, see the "Seizures" entry in this section.)

Reye's syndrome

Fatty degeneration of the viscera and acute encephalopathy, often occurring after an acute viral infection.

NURSING DIAGNOSIS

Anxiety (parental) related to the uncertainty of the disorder's outcome

DESIRED PATIENT OUTCOME

The parents will demonstrate reduced anxiety about the child's condition

Outcome measurement criteria

- ☐ Verbalization by the parents of reduced anxiety
- ☐ Description by the parents of previous coping patterns
- ☐ Participation of the parents in the child's care when feasible
- ☐ Demonstration by family members of support for one another
- ☐ Use of community support systems
- ☐ Verbalization by the parents of increased comfort with the situation

Key interventions

- Encourage the parents to express their concerns about the child's disorder and its outcome.
- Encourage the parents to describe previously successful coping techniques. Help them apply those techniques in this situation.
- Explain treatments and update the parents frequently on the child's care and responses to care.

- Permit the parents to stay with the child as much as possible.
- Facilitate the parents' and other family members' involvement in the child's care, when feasible, assuring them that the child will be well cared for when family members are absent.
- Encourage the extended family to provide support, such as caring for other children, staying with the child when the parents must be absent, and helping with household tasks.
- Refer the parents to appropriate community support groups and agencies.

NURSING DIAGNOSIS

High risk for injury related to the effects of Reye's syndrome

DESIRED PATIENT OUTCOME

The child will sustain no injuries because of the syndrome's effects

Outcome measurement criteria

- ☐ Normal neurologic signs
- ☐ Normal aspartate aminotransferase (AST), alanine aminotransferase (ALT), and ammonia levels
- ☐ Age-appropriate intracranial pressure (ICP)
- ☐ Age-appropriate urine output and urine specific gravity
- ☐ Patent airway
- ☐ Normal vital signs
- ☐ Arterial blood gas (ABG), serum pH, and serum electrolyte values within normal ranges
- ☐ Normal blood glucose level
- ☐ Intact skin

☐ Clotting test results within normal limits

☐ Normal gag, swallow, and blink reflexes

Key interventions

- Record neurologic checks and the stage of neurologic involvement every hour. Notify the primary care practitioner of deterioration.
- Report abnormal AST, ALT, and ammonia levels to the primary care practitioner.
- Monitor for increased ICP, calculate cerebral perfusion pressure, and notify the primary care practitioner of an abrupt increase or serial increases in ICP.
- Elevate the head of the bed to 30 degrees, maintain the child's head in the midline position, and minimize stimuli, such as noise, light, touch, and pain.
- Administer medications as prescribed to help keep ICP within the normal range.
- Administer I.V. solution exactly as prescribed and maintain strict fluid intake and output records. Notify the primary care practitioner if output is less than 1 ml/kg/hour.
- Perform indwelling urinary catheter care and check urine specific gravity every 2 hours.
- Maintain a patent airway, suctioning only if essential and hyperventilating the child before and after suctioning; record the character of secretions. Administer prescribed medications to maintain intubation.
- Auscultate the chest every 2 hours and monitor pulse and respiratory rates and blood pressure. Notify the primary care practitioner of abnormal findings.
- Monitor ABG, pH, and electrolyte values. Notify the primary care practitioner if abnormal values do not respond to interventions.

- Inspect the skin while providing other care. Coordinate care to minimize stimulation, gently perform range-of-motion exercises and turning if ICP is within the normal range, use an egg-crate mattress cover, and note signs of bleeding.
- Monitor prothrombin time, partial thromboplastin time, and platelet count. Report abnormal values to the primary care practitioner.
- Assess for gag and swallow reflexes. Monitor for the blink reflex. If the reflex is absent, keep the child's eyelids closed and instill the prescribed eye lubricant.
- Take seizure precautions. (For details, see the "Seizures" entry in this section.)

Seizures

Abnormal electrical activity in the brain that causes transient, recurrent, involuntary movements that range from mild localized muscle twitching to severe generalized muscle contraction and relaxation, and behaviors that range from staring to loss of consciousness.

NURSING DIAGNOSIS

Altered protection related to seizures

DESIRED PATIENT OUTCOME

The child will sustain no injuries during seizures

Outcome measurement criteria

- ☐ Inclusion by the nurse of safety measures in the care plan
- ☐ Removal by the nurse and parents of potentially dangerous objects from the environment
- ☐ Absence of aspiration by the child
- ☐ Absence of injury to the child due to hitting hard surfaces
- ☐ Accurate report by the parents of seizure activity
- ☐ Age-appropriate body temperature of the child
- ☐ Administration by the parents of prescribed medications
- ☐ Attendance by the parents and child at follow-up visits

Key interventions

- Discuss with the parents the potential for seizures and explain the reasons for safety precautions.

- Assess the child's environment for situations and objects that might cause injury.
- Remove from the child's crib (if applicable) and room objects that could cause harm during seizures.
- Keep crib or bed side rails up.
- Teach the parents to place the child on the side during seizures; to carefully document seizure activity, noting any aura and the duration, location, and movements associated with the seizure; to notify the primary care practitioner of seizure activity; to monitor the child's body temperature and use prescribed medication and a cooling atmosphere to lower the temperature as needed; to notify the primary care practitioner if the temperature remains elevated; to administer seizure medications and monitor the child for adverse effects; and to make appointments with the primary care practitioner to monitor the child's seizure medication levels and general growth and development.

NURSING DIAGNOSIS

High risk for social isolation related to fear of having a seizure

DESIRED PATIENT OUTCOME

The child will maintain social interactions with family members and friends

Outcome measurement criteria

- ☐ Verbalization of feelings about having a seizure
- ☐ Verbalization of willingness to participate in social interactions
- ☐ Participation in activities that the child enjoys
- ☐ Identification of ways to increase social interactions

Key interventions

- Discuss with the child feelings about having seizures. Determine the child's stage of grief and degree of adjustment to the problem.
- Explore, if age appropriate, the child's willingness to participate in social situations. Help the child analyze the advantages and disadvantages of social involvement.
- Have the child describe social activities that are enjoyable, discussing which activities are feasible considering the child's disorder.
- Discuss ways to increase age-appropriate and physically feasible social activities.

Anorexia nervosa or bulimia nervosa

Eating disorders characterized by extreme anxiety about weight gain and caused by a pervasive sense of lack of control over one's life. Anorexia nervosa is characterized by weight loss due to self-imposed restricted food intake and can lead to emaciation if not treated. Bulimia nervosa is characterized by repeated food binges followed by GI tract purging by induced vomiting or laxative abuse.

NURSING DIAGNOSIS

Altered nutrition: less than body requirements, related to aversion to weight gain or self-induced vomiting and laxative abuse

DESIRED PATIENT OUTCOME

The child will maintain age-appropriate nutrient and food intake

Outcome measurement criteria

- ☐ Verbalization by the child of an understanding that inappropriate eating behaviors are unhealthy and dangerous
- ☐ Age-appropriate nutrient and food intake
- ☐ Age-appropriate vital signs and activity level
- ☐ Attainment of goal weight as determined by the child and the health care team
- ☐ Laboratory test values reflecting adequate nutrition
- ☐ Absence of binging and purging

Key interventions

- Discuss with the child the physiological effects of malnutrition.
- Consult with a dietitian and develop a plan with the child and the health care team to meet the child's nutritional needs.
- Involve the child in planning a diet that includes frequent, small meals rather than three large meals and provide the child's favorite high-protein, high-carbohydrate foods.
- Provide nutritious snacks, such as high-protein shakes.
- Observe the child closely during meals to determine intake and after meals to detect purging.
- Monitor fecal output for evidence of laxative use.
- Monitor vital signs and activity level for signs of poor nutrition.
- Develop a contract with the child that provides rewards for compliance and removes privileges for noncompliance. Arrange for the child to be tube-fed if weight loss continues.
- Weigh the child early each morning after the child has voided, using the same scale and with the child wearing the same amount of clothing. Remind the child that weight gain will be slow. Work with the child to set a target weight for discharge.
- Monitor the results of laboratory tests, including blood chemistry studies. Report abnormal values to the primary care practitioner.
- Develop a system in which the child can get help when tempted to binge, induce vomiting, or take laxatives.
- Avoid judgmental comments; focus on the child's feelings.
- Assess the child for depression, suicide risk, and anxiety.

NURSING DIAGNOSIS

Body image disturbance related to perception of self as obese

DESIRED PATIENT OUTCOME

The child will perceive body size accurately

Outcome measurement criteria

- ☐ Verbalization by the child of positive, realistic feelings about the body
- ☐ Verbalization by the child of appropriate ways to achieve control over problematic aspects of life
- ☐ Participation in therapy by the family

Key interventions

- Develop a trusting relationship with the family.
- Help the child gain a realistic perception of body size. Compare the child's body weight with norms based on age, sex, and frame and with those of another child of the same age and sex.
- Encourage participation in group sessions, and use techniques that encourage a positive self-image.
- Encourage the child to discuss perceived personal strengths and weaknesses; help dismiss unfounded self-criticism and misconceptions.
- Explore with the child the aspects of life over which the child feels a lack of control. Discuss whether controlling these aspects is realistic and, if so, to what degree. Help the child identify ways to achieve control over these aspects by assessing personal strengths and the support of others.
- Suggest alternative methods of coping with stress.
- Provide the family with therapy opportunities.
- Observe and document family interactions.

Autism, infantile

Syndrome of early childhood characterized by failure to develop social relationships, developmental language disorders, repetitive behaviors and, often, retarded intellectual development.

NURSING DIAGNOSIS

Impaired social interaction related to the effects of autism

DESIRED PATIENT OUTCOME

The child will interact with the parents and other caregivers

Outcome measurement criteria

- ☐ Eye contact with the parents and other caregivers
- ☐ Use of means of communication
- ☐ Appropriate interactions with others

Key interventions

- Establish a trusting relationship with the child.
- Reward the child with praise and treats for making eye contact.
- Use a play therapist to encourage communication.
- Find a way to communicate with the child that minimizes the child's frustration, such as matching pictures with words. Reward the child for appropriate communication.
- Assess the child's usual interactions and develop a plan to modify interactions so they are more socially acceptable.

NURSING DIAGNOSIS

High risk for self-mutilation related to the effects of autism

DESIRED PATIENT OUTCOME

The child will not harm self

Outcome measurement criteria

- ☐ Use of means of communication
- ☐ Eye contact with caregivers
- ☐ Absence of self-mutilation

Key interventions

- Establish a trusting relationship with the child.
- Establish a way to communicate with the child; anticipate the need to decrease the child's frustration.
- Determine which events precipitate self-mutilating behavior, and try to prevent them from occurring.
- Provide the child with alternative ways to communicate frustration and anger.
- Praise the child for non-self-mutilating behavior. Establish eye contact when giving praise and provide a reward.
- Apply protective devices, such as a helmet or padded arm and leg covers, to prevent self-mutilation.

Child abuse or neglect

Maltreatment of a child or failure to provide adequate care for the child.

NURSING DIAGNOSIS

Fear (child) related to removal from the parents

DESIRED PATIENT OUTCOME

The child will demonstrate psychological comfort

Outcome measurement criteria

☐ Verbalization of fears (if age-appropriate)

☐ Open communication (if age-appropriate) with health care personnel

Key interventions

- Establish a trusting relationship with the child, assigning consistent caregivers.
- Demonstrate kindness toward and acceptance of the child.
- Encourage the child to express anxieties and fears; use a play therapist to help the child verbalize feelings (if age-appropriate).
- Tell the child (if age-appropriate) that the interview is confidential and use language that the child understands.
- Accurately record the child's statements (if age-appropriate) that explain maltreatment or lack of care. Ask the child to explain words you do not understand.

NURSING DIAGNOSIS

Ineffective individual coping (nonabusing parent) related to fear of the abuser

DESIRED PATIENT OUTCOME

The nonabusing parent will interrupt the child abuser's behavior

Outcome measurement criteria

- ☐ Verbalization by the nonabusing parent to outsiders of the child abuser's behavior
- ☐ Description by the nonabusing parent of details of abuse, for documentation purposes
- ☐ Prevention of child abuse by the nonabusing parent

Key interventions

- Build a trusting relationship with the nonabusing parent and other family members.
- Encourage the nonabusing parent to discuss the abusive behaviors and feelings about the situation.
- Record details of abuse in the parent's words.
- Develop a plan with the nonabusing parent to remove the child from the abuser's presence.
- Facilitate the nonabusing parent's use of community agencies to relocate to a safe place with the child.
- If the nonabusing parent refuses to remove the child from the abusive situation, explain the legal responsibility of nurses to contact a state agency responsible for protecting children.

NURSING DIAGNOSIS

Ineffective family coping: disabling, related to situational factors

DESIRED PATIENT OUTCOME

The family will function effectively as a unit

Outcome measurement criteria

- ☐ Verbalization by family members of their problems and need for assistance
- ☐ Identification by family members of factors that contribute to ineffective family functioning and abuse
- ☐ Use by the family of community resources
- ☐ Demonstration by family members of mutual support

Key interventions

- Help the family openly discuss their problems.
- Listen for complaints about the child by the parents.
- Assess the parents' responses and attitudes toward the child, noting the way each parent holds and touches the child.
- Discuss events that precede incidents of child abuse.
- Discuss the parents' expectations of the child.
- Discourage the parents from blaming the child, but allow them to vent feelings.
- Develop a plan to use when abuse seems imminent, such as calling a hotline, other family members, a support group member, a social worker, legal services, or a shelter.
- Assess for signs of parental conflict or lack of mutual support, which can lead to an abusive incident.

NURSING DIAGNOSIS

High risk for altered health maintenance related to insufficient parenting skills

DESIRED PATIENT OUTCOME

The parents will effectively maintain the child's health

Outcome measurement criteria

- ☐ Verbalization by the parents of realistic, age-appropriate expectations of the child
- ☐ Identification by the parents of aspects of health maintenance with which they need assistance
- ☐ Use of a plan by the parents to promote their development of health maintenance skills
- ☐ Consistent attendance at parenting skills sessions
- ☐ Use by the parents of community supports

Key interventions

- Explore the parents' expectations of the child. Discuss whether these expectations are realistic and why.
- Determine which parenting skills the parents need help with. Model parenting skills when in the presence of the child and parents.
- Develop a plan to provide continual assistance with and evaluation of parenting skills, involving parenting skills sessions and community supports.
- Determine the need for immediate services, such as hotlines, respite programs, and weekend relief.

Depression

Emotional state characterized by extreme sadness, despair, worthlessness, and hopelessness.

NURSING DIAGNOSIS

Ineffective individual coping related to low self-esteem and situational stressors

DESIRED PATIENT OUTCOME

The child will demonstrate effective coping skills

Outcome measurement criteria

- ☐ Verbalization of a realistic self-perception
- ☐ Identification of positive aspects of self
- ☐ Participation in positive social interactions and activities
- ☐ Demonstration of appropriate mood and behavior
- ☐ Identification of effective strategies for coping with situational stressors

Key interventions

- Develop a trusting relationship with the child, communicating with the child in an age-appropriate, caring manner.
- Encourage the child to discuss feelings about the self and help the child identify positive aspects of personality.
- Involve the child in routine self-care, such as hygiene, dressing, and eating with a group.
- Praise the child when appearance is improved.

- Provide daily physical exercise.
- Expect the child to visit the activity area and encourage the child to participate in structured group activities.
- Encourage the child to interact with others.
- Assess the child's mood and behavior.
- Observe and document family interactions that indicate dysfunctional family patterns.
- Teach the family effective coping techniques and refer them for counseling, if indicated.

NURSING DIAGNOSIS

High risk for social isolation related to feelings of hopelessness and worthlessness

DESIRED PATIENT OUTCOME

The child will interact appropriately with peers

Outcome measurement criteria

- ☐ Verbalization by the child of positive aspects of self
- ☐ Identification by the child of factors that deter or prevent social interaction
- ☐ Participation by the child in social activities
- ☐ Absence of acting-out behaviors

Key interventions

- Develop a trusting relationship with the child, communicating in an age-appropriate manner and demonstrating a caring attitude.
- Encourage the child to discuss perceived personal strengths and weaknesses. Help the child dispel misconceptions about the self and reinforce the child's strengths.

- Identify factors that hinder social interaction and promote the child's social activities.
- Teach the child helpful social skills, such as assertiveness, nonjudgmental attitude, and communication skills. Have the child try out these skills in a small, supportive group.
- Encourage the child to seek out interesting group activities at church or school or in the community.
- Recognize the child's efforts to interact; if the child becomes anxious in a group, let the child leave to reduce anxiety.
- Administer medication as prescribed. Explain its therapeutic and adverse effects to the parents and child, and identify foods to avoid when taking a monoamine oxidase (MAO) inhibitor.

NURSING DIAGNOSIS

High risk for altered nutrition: less than body requirements, related to inappropriate eating patterns

DESIRED PATIENT OUTCOME

The child will maintain age-appropriate nutrient and food intake

Outcome measurement criteria

- ☐ Age-appropriate vital signs, particularly temperature
- ☐ Age-appropriate weight and nutrient intake
- ☐ Elastic skin turgor
- ☐ Hemoglobin, hematocrit, and blood chemistry values within normal limits

Key interventions

- Assess vital signs daily, closely monitoring the child's temperature.
- Weigh the child daily at same time, on the same scale, and with the child wearing the same amount of clothing; compare the child's weight to age-group norms.
- Assess eating patterns and monitor food and fluid intake. However, do not pressure the child to eat.
- Involve the child in choosing and preparing foods. Teach the family the foods to avoid if the child is taking an MAO inhibitor.
- Provide small meals, between-meal snacks, and prescribed vitamins or nutritional supplements.
- Check the child's skin turgor if fluid intake is inadequate.
- Monitor hemoglobin, hematocrit, and blood chemistry values. Notify the primary care practitioner if values are abnormal.

NURSING DIAGNOSIS

Sleep pattern disturbance related to emotional stress

DESIRED PATIENT OUTCOME

The child will display age-appropriate sleep patterns

Outcome measurement criteria

☐ Age-appropriate amount of nightly sleep

☐ Establishment of a bedtime routine

☐ Establishment of a daytime sleep limit

Key interventions

- Assess the child's sleep patterns. Ask about difficulty falling asleep, nighttime awakening, nonrestful sleep, and excessive sleep, determining the number of hours the child sleeps each night. Find out if the child has a bedtime routine and if it is conducive to sleep.
- Establish the expectation that the child will go to bed and arise at specified times. Discourage daytime sleeping.
- Provide relaxation measures at bedtime and remove sources of stimulation, such as television and radio. Develop a bedtime routine if the child does not have one.

NURSING DIAGNOSIS

High risk for violence: self-directed, related to situational factors

DESIRED PATIENT OUTCOME

The child will not injure self intentionally

Outcome measurement criteria

- ☐ Absence of self-inflicted harm
- ☐ Verbalization by the child of feelings
- ☐ Identification by the child of factors that contribute to feelings of worthlessness
- ☐ Identification by the child of effective coping techniques
- ☐ Use by the family of a protective plan to prevent the child from self-harm
- ☐ Acceptance by the child of help from others in dealing with feelings and life situations

Key interventions

- Ask if the child has thought about committing suicide and, if so, when and how; ask about previous suicide attempts.
- Ask why the child considered suicide, including what events occurred and what feelings were present.
- Discuss alternative ways to deal with events and feelings that make the child consider suicide.
- Help the child recall previously successful coping techniques.
- Provide a safe environment so that the child cannot cause self-harm. Supervise the child closely, follow health care facility policy, and inform staff members and visitors of the child's wish to inflict self-harm so they will not unknowingly contribute to the plan. Remove potentially lethal objects from the child's environment, and supervise the taking of medications so the child cannot stockpile them.
- Develop a "no suicide" contract with the child, in which the child agrees to tell the staff when thoughts and feelings of self-harm occur; praise the child's efforts to protect the self by seeking assistance.
- Develop a "no harm" contract when the child is discharged, involving the parents and child in the contract. Teach the parents signs of potential self-harm, and give the parents and child the telephone numbers to call for immediate assistance if needed.
- Observe and document positive and maladaptive family functioning.
- Provide therapy for the family, and encourage them to use community support systems, such as church, community groups, and health care facility–based support groups.

Failure to thrive, inorganic

Retardation or cessation of growth and development because of nonphysiologic factors.

NURSING DIAGNOSIS

Altered parenting related to lack of knowledge about parenting skills

DESIRED PATIENT OUTCOME

The parents will demonstrate appropriate parenting skills

Outcome measurement criteria

- ☐ Development by the parents and nurse of a plan to promote parenting skills
- ☐ Consistent attendance at parenting skills sessions
- ☐ Verbalization by the parents of realistic, age-appropriate expectations of the child

Key interventions

- Determine if the parents fit a category—such as adolescent, mentally retarded, or older parents—to help determine an appropriate approach.
- Assess the parents' ability to care for the child's needs, such as feeding, bathing, communicating, and giving emotional support.
- Create a plan with the parents to systematically develop parenting skills if many skills are lacking.
- Use role modeling to teach the parents the skills they lack. Answer their questions, clarify points, acknowledge skills the parents possess, and reinforce positive parenting abilities.

- Encourage the parents to attend parenting skill sessions by creating a pleasant and rewarding atmosphere and by positively reinforcing the parents' efforts.
- Provide information on normal growth and development, and help the parents learn realistic, age-appropriate norms for the child.

NURSING DIAGNOSIS

Altered nutrition: less than body requirements, related to inadequate food intake

DESIRED PATIENT OUTCOME

The child will maintain age-appropriate nutrient and food intake

Outcome measurement criteria

- ☐ Verbalization by the parents of the child's need for adequate nutrition
- ☐ Demonstration by the parents of appropriate feeding techniques
- ☐ Age-appropriate weight and nutrient intake
- ☐ Elastic skin turgor
- ☐ Hemoglobin, hematocrit, and blood chemistry values within normal limits
- ☐ Age-appropriate growth and development

Key interventions

- Assess the parents' knowledge about nutrition. Discuss the child's need for nutrients and fluids for growth and development.
- Assess the parents' feeding techniques, demonstrate appropriate feeding methods, and positively reinforce the parents' use of proper techniques.

- Weigh the child early each morning after the child has voided, using the same scale and with the child wearing the same amount of clothing.
- Document all food and fluid intake to estimate the child's consumption; offer high-protein, high-calorie foods between meals; and determine the child's response to food.
- Assess skin turgor.
- Monitor hemoglobin, hematocrit, and blood chemistry values. Notify the primary care practitioner about abnormal values.
- Administer the Denver II Developmental Screening Test to assess developmental status. Promote the parents' use of community agencies to assist the child in correcting developmental delays.

Mental retardation

Disorder in which the child has less-than-average intelligence, resulting in an inability to function fully in society.

NURSING DIAGNOSIS

Grieving (parental) related to loss of the child's mental health

DESIRED PATIENT OUTCOME

The parents will cope effectively with their grief at the loss of the child's mental health

Outcome measurement criteria

- ☐ Expression of grief by the parents
- ☐ Verbalization by the parents that reflects an understanding of grieving
- ☐ Demonstration of mutual support by family members
- ☐ Verbalization by the parents of a plan to deal with the immediate details of the child's care

Key interventions

- Assess the parents' past experiences with grief and loss.
- Explain that grief is normal, clarify the stages of grieving, and correct misconceptions.
- Identify the family's strengths as a unit and as individuals.
- Encourage discussion of the parents' feelings about the child's mental retardation.
- Encourage the parents to be open and truthful with other family members, including the child.

- Prepare the parents for the possible responses of others to the child's mental retardation.
- Discuss ways for the parents to handle the immediate details of the child's care, such as providing adequate care for the child and siblings, making special arrangements with employers, making financial arrangements for the child's care, and modifying the home environment, as needed.

NURSING DIAGNOSIS

Anxiety related to lack of knowledge about mental retardation

DESIRED PATIENT OUTCOME

The family and child (if developmentally appropriate) will demonstrate increased knowledge and reduced anxiety about the child's condition

Outcome measurement criteria

- ☐ Verbalization by the family of accurate knowledge about mental retardation
- ☐ Verbalization by the family of the effects of mental retardation on the child and family as a unit and as individuals
- ☐ Use by the family of community support systems for learning about mental retardation
- ☐ Participation by the family and child, if feasible, in the child's care
- ☐ Return of the child and family members to their usual eating and sleeping patterns and developmental tasks
- ☐ Continued child growth and development, to the degree the condition permits
- ☐ Verbalization by family members of increased comfort with the child's condition

□ Involvement of the family in a support group

Key interventions

- Assess the family's knowledge about mental retardation.
- Teach the family about the child's mental retardation.
- Encourage the siblings to use play to act out anxiety and fear.
- Encourage open communication among family members and between the nurse and family members.
- Encourage discussions by the family about the effects of mental retardation on the family's lifestyle.
- Plan how the child, if able, and each family member can contribute to the child's care.
- Demonstrate how to provide the special care the child needs.
- Support and provide positive feedback to the family as they learn aspects of care.
- Periodically assess the child's and family members' eating and sleeping patterns and developmental tasks, including play (for the child and siblings). Also, regularly assess the child's growth and development.
- Urge the family to become involved with a support group.

NURSING DIAGNOSIS

High risk for feeding, bathing, hygiene, dressing, and grooming self-care deficits related to impaired cognitive functioning

DESIRED PATIENT OUTCOME

The parents and child (if developmentally appropriate) will meet the child's self-care needs

Outcome measurement criteria

- ☐ Verbalization by the parents of feelings about the child's self-care limitations
- ☐ Demonstration by the parents and child (if developmentally appropriate) of competence in meeting the child's self-care needs
- ☐ Verbalization by the parents of positive feelings about adapting to the child's self-care limitations
- ☐ Use of a health care team to help meet the child's self-care needs
- ☐ Use of community resources to help meet the child's self-care needs

Key interventions

- Encourage the family to discuss feelings about the child's inability to meet specific self-care needs.
- Demonstrate alternative ways to meet the child's self-care needs.
- Encourage the family to allow the child to perform or assist with self-care, if feasible.
- Assemble a health care team to help the family meet the child's specific self-care needs.
- Identify community support systems that the family can use to help meet the child's specific self-care needs.
- Discuss ways to obtain financial assistance to meet the child's special needs.
- Encourage the family to meet with other families in similar circumstances.

NURSING DIAGNOSIS

High risk for caregiver role strain related to the demands of caring for a mentally retarded child

DESIRED PATIENT OUTCOME

The family will adjust effectively to caring for the mentally retarded child

Outcome measurement criteria

- ☐ Demonstration by family members of affection for the child
- ☐ Open expression of feelings by the parents and siblings
- ☐ Open and appropriate communication among family members
- ☐ Demonstration by family members of mutual support
- ☐ Use by the parents of specific community support systems to help meet the family's and child's needs
- ☐ Participation by the family in the child's care
- ☐ Fulfillment by the family of the child's health care needs
- ☐ Achievement by the child of modified developmental milestones and appropriate social development
- ☐ Identification by the parents of specific stressors
- ☐ Use by the parents of a plan to counter stress
- ☐ Verbalization by the parents of increased control over the situation

Key interventions

- Obtain thorough family and child health histories, assessing the family's strengths and weaknesses and the child's physical needs and developmental status.
- Encourage family members to discuss feelings openly.
- Explore the family's feelings of guilt, anger, sadness, and hopelessness and ways to deal with them.
- Encourage the family to use community support systems.

- Have the family plan and share care for the child, including physical, psychosocial, and developmental aspects of care.
- Identify coping techniques that family members have used successfully in previous family crises.
- Identify stressful aspects of having a mentally retarded child, such as the child's need for long-term treatment outside the home and special schooling, financial demands, reactions of siblings and friends, decreased social opportunities for family members, difficulty in obtaining a baby-sitter, too little time for the parents as a couple and as individuals, and anxiety about the child's long-term care.
- Develop a plan to minimize stress in family members. Help the parents plan time for each sibling to receive special attention each week; encourage the parents to set limits for the child similar to those imposed on siblings; and help the parents obtain respite care.

Obesity

Body weight greater than 20% above normal for a person's height and body frame.

NURSING DIAGNOSIS

Ineffective individual coping related to increased food consumption

DESIRED PATIENT OUTCOME

The child will substitute effective coping techniques for eating

Outcome measurement criteria

- ☐ Verbalization of feelings about obesity
- ☐ Identification of events that precipitate increased food consumption
- ☐ Identification of personal strengths and successful coping techniques for dealing with problems
- ☐ Acceptance of help from other persons or groups

Key interventions

- Develop a trusting relationship with the child.
- Discuss feelings about the child's obesity.
- Discuss events that precipitate increased food consumption, assess for symptoms of depression, and explore perceived losses that may contribute to the child's obesity.
- Encourage the child to discuss perceived personal strengths and weaknesses and dismiss unfounded self-criticism and misconceptions. Explore previously successful coping techniques.

- Explore aspects of life over which the child feels a lack of control, and help the child determine healthy ways to achieve control over major aspects of life.
- Explore alternative techniques for coping with stress, such as art, dancing, and other activities.
- Observe and document maladaptive family functioning.
- Refer the family for counseling, if indicated.
- Promote the parents' and child's use of support groups.

NURSING DIAGNOSIS

Altered health maintenance related to lack of knowledge about exercise and diet

DESIRED PATIENT OUTCOME

The parents and child (if age-appropriate) will demonstrate an understanding of age-appropriate exercise and diet

Outcome measurement criteria

- ☐ Verbalization by the parents and child (if age-appropriate) of age-appropriate exercise and play
- ☐ Verbalization by the parents and child (if age-appropriate) of age-appropriate diet
- ☐ Participation by the parents and child (if age-appropriate) in planning the child's diet
- ☐ Age-appropriate food and fluid intake and body weight

Key interventions

- Teach the parents and child (if age-appropriate) the physiological effects of obesity.

- Consult with an exercise physiologist, develop a plan to meet the child's exercise needs, and provide an opportunity for the child to meet with a support group of similar-age children.
- Encourage the parents to provide opportunities for daily active play and exercise, using church, community, and school groups, when possible.
- Consult with a dietitian and develop a plan to meet the child's nutritional needs. With the child, develop a contract that rewards compliance with the diet plan.
- Involve the child in preparing menus, using low-fat and favorite foods as much as possible. Provide nutritious, low-fat snacks. Encourage the parents to model appropriate eating behaviors.
- Weigh the child weekly after the child has voided, using the same scale and with the child wearing the same amount of clothing.

NURSING DIAGNOSIS

High risk for social isolation related to fear of negative responses from others

DESIRED PATIENT OUTCOME

The child will interact appropriately with peers

Outcome measurement criteria

- ☐ Verbalization by the child of positive aspects of personality and appearance
- ☐ Verbalization by the child of feelings about social situations
- ☐ Participation by the child in group social activities

Key interventions

- Establish a trusting relationship with the child. Use age-appropriate language and communicate a caring attitude.
- Encourage the child to discuss perceived strengths and weaknesses. Dispel misconceptions about the self and reinforce the child's strengths.
- Determine factors that hinder social interaction and promote the child's social activities.
- Teach the child helpful social skills, such as communication skills.
- Praise the child's efforts to be socially interactive.

Schizophrenia

Mental disorder characterized by psychotic symptoms, including disturbances in thought processes, feelings, and behavior.

NURSING DIAGNOSIS

Impaired verbal communication related to the effects of schizophrenia and its treatment

DESIRED PATIENT OUTCOME

The child will communicate appropriately and effectively

Outcome measurement criteria

- ☐ Ability to express thoughts in an age-appropriate manner
- ☐ Verbalization of reality-based ideas
- ☐ Use of medication that does not impair communication

Key interventions

- Use consistent caregivers for the child as much as possible. Build a trusting, caring relationship with the child. Be sincere, empathetic, honest, and consistent in dealing with the child.
- Anticipate and meet the child's needs when the child is communicating ineffectively.
- Call the child by name. Avoid touching the child, which can precipitate a violent response.
- Clarify and validate communicated messages. Tell the child when a message is not understood, but do not argue with the child or question the content of the message.

- Respond to the child in an age-appropriate and accepting manner. Communicate the reality of situations.
- Administer medications as prescribed and document their effects on the child.
- Notify the primary care practitioner if the child experiences adverse effects or extreme sleepiness or if behavior is unimproved.
- Explain to the parents and child that the child should take the prescribed medications even when feeling well. Teach them about the medications' adverse effects.

NURSING DIAGNOSIS

Impaired social interaction related to the effects of schizophrenia

DESIRED PATIENT OUTCOME

The child will interact appropriately with peers

Outcome measurement criteria

- ☐ Verbalization by the child of positive aspects of the self
- ☐ Identification by the nurse and child of factors that promote or prevent the child's social interactions
- ☐ Development of a plan by the nurse and child of ways to reduce social limitations and promote social relationships
- ☐ Verbalization or role-playing by the child of positive social interactions
- ☐ Participation by the child in individual and group social relationships
- ☐ Compliance by the child with the medication regimen

Key interventions

- Establish a trusting relationship with the child. Use age-appropriate language and communicate a caring attitude.
- Encourage the child to discuss perceived personal strengths and weaknesses. Dispel misconceptions and reinforce strengths.
- Discuss factors that hinder social interaction and promote the child's social activities. Encourage the child to discuss and role-play social interactions and then to participate in social relationships.
- Praise the child's efforts to be socially interactive; record the effects of groups on the child's ability to remain socially active.
- Administer medications as prescribed, explaining their therapeutic and adverse effects to the parents and child.

Asthma

Obstructive respiratory disease caused by excessive reaction of the airway to various stimuli, resulting in narrowed airway passages and increased bronchial mucus and characterized by coughing, dyspnea, and wheezing.

NURSING DIAGNOSIS

High risk for ineffective breathing pattern related to lack of knowledge about asthma and its management

DESIRED PATIENT OUTCOME

The parents and child (if age-appropriate) will prevent or reduce the severity of asthmatic attacks

Outcome measurement criteria

- ☐ Identification by the parents and child (if age-appropriate) of factors that trigger attacks
- ☐ Verbalization by the parents and child (if age-appropriate) of signs and symptoms of an impending asthma attack
- ☐ Verbalization by the parents and child (if age-appropriate) of measures to take if an attack seems imminent or begins
- ☐ Modification of the home, particularly the child's bedroom and play area
- ☐ Demonstration by the parents and child (if age-appropriate) of correct hand-washing technique
- ☐ Age-appropriate diet and avoidance of known food allergens

- ☐ Age-appropriate exercise and play
- ☐ Absence of signs and symptoms of infection
- ☐ Daily fluid intake of six to eight 8-ounce (240-ml) glasses
- ☐ Absence of respiratory distress, including dyspnea
- ☐ Absence of extensive physical or emotional stress

Key interventions

- Teach the parents and child (if age-appropriate) to identify factors that trigger attacks, such as allergens, infections, exercise, stress, and smoke. Remove unnecessary decorations and carpeting. Wet-mop the floor daily and wash walls regularly. Avoid plants, aquariums, and other mold and mildew sources; wool and other allergenic fabrics; animals; smoking areas; and stuffed toys. Close the windows during allergy seasons.
- Reduce exposure to infection by having the child avoid crowds during cold and flu season and practice good hygiene and hand-washing technique.
- Teach the parents how to provide an age-appropriate diet, avoiding allergenic food.
- Reduce stress by providing opportunities for appropriate play and exercise, encouraging open communication between the parents and child, and teaching relaxation techniques.
- Teach the parents and child (if age-appropriate) the warning signs of an asthma attack, including an itchy chin or throat, fatigue, headache, chest tightness, glassy eyes, nasal drainage, and irritability.
- Teach the parents and child (if age-appropriate) immediate care if an attack seems imminent or begins, including starting prescribed medications, drinking fluids for adequate hydration, resting in a comfortable position, using relaxation techniques, checking oral temperature and notifying the primary care practitioner

if the temperature is over 99° F (37.2° C), checking for signs of infection, using aerosol equipment if indicated, and visiting the primary care practitioner or the emergency department if the attack worsens.

NURSING DIAGNOSIS

Ineffective breathing pattern related to increased mucus production and narrowed respiratory passages

DESIRED PATIENT OUTCOME

The child will display an effective breathing pattern

Outcome measurement criteria

- ☐ Identification by the parents and child (if age-appropriate) of events that provoke or relieve asthma attacks
- ☐ Absence of chest retractions, wheezing, rhonchi, or accessory muscle use
- ☐ Normal color in lips and nail beds
- ☐ Normal pulse and respiratory rates
- ☐ Arterial blood gas (ABG) levels within normal range
- ☐ Age-appropriate urine output and urine specific gravity
- ☐ Elastic skin turgor
- ☐ Moist mucous membranes

Key interventions

- Obtain a history of the onset of attacks and medications taken.
- Administer epinephrine, as prescribed, for acute respiratory distress. If epinephrine is ineffective, administer aminophylline, as prescribed, using an infusion pump.
- Monitor serum theophylline levels and assess for signs of toxicity, such as vomiting, irritability, and tachycardia.

- Monitor for the effects of medications every 30 to 60 minutes during the acute phase.
- Administer aerosol treatments and repeat as prescribed. Administer oxygen at the prescribed rate.
- Monitor I.V. fluids and the I.V. site.
- Offer small sips of favorite clear liquids.
- Observe for signs of dehydration, such as vital sign changes, poor skin turgor, dry mucosa, sunken eyes, decreased urine output, and elevated urine specific gravity.
- Monitor vital signs every 15 minutes for 1 to 2 hours.
- Auscultate breath sounds and observe the child's facial expression and body position. Place the child in an upright, relaxed position.
- Check lip and nail bed color.
- Assess ABG levels.
- Note nasal flaring and chest retractions.
- Teach the parents and child how to administer medications correctly.
- Teach the parents and child how to use the inhaler, nebulizer, and other breathing equipment.
- Teach breathing exercises and effective coughing and expectoration.

NURSING DIAGNOSIS

High risk for caregiver role strain related to the stress of caring for a chronically ill child

DESIRED PATIENT OUTCOME

The family members will successfully cope with the effects of the child's disease on family life and will promote normal development

Outcome measurement criteria

- ☐ Seeking and acceptance by the family of assistance
- ☐ Verbalization by family members of feelings
- ☐ Open and effective communication among family members
- ☐ Meeting by family members of their biopsychosocial needs
- ☐ Verbalization by family members of realistic expectations of the child
- ☐ Verbalization by the child of a positive self-image

Key interventions

- Assist the family in using appropriate support systems.
- Help the family seek financial assistance as needed.
- Encourage family members to communicate openly and verbalize feelings, such as guilt, anger, frustration, depression, and anxiety.
- Encourage individual activities and activities in which all family members can participate.
- Promote the child's development by encouraging age-appropriate activities, unless contraindicated.
- Provide opportunities for the child to succeed at activities appropriate to the child's physical condition.
- Monitor family members for manipulative or maladaptive behavior and intervene appropriately. Help family members develop realistic expectations of the child and help the child develop a positive self-image.

Bronchopulmonary dysplasia

Chronic lung disease caused by long-term, intensive therapy for severe respiratory problems in infants.

NURSING DIAGNOSIS

Impaired gas exchange related to the effects of bronchopulmonary dysplasia (BPD)

DESIRED PATIENT OUTCOME

The child will display appropriate gas exchange

Outcome measurement criteria

- ☐ Age-appropriate and condition-appropriate oxygen and carbon dioxide levels
- ☐ Absence of respiratory infection
- ☐ Absence of excessive mucus in airway

Key interventions

- Monitor oxygen and carbon dioxide levels according to health care facility protocol, using the smallest amount of oxygen needed to maintain adequate oxygen levels.
- Check and document ventilator settings according to health care facility policy—usually every hour.
- Assess vital signs by monitoring continuously or at least hourly. Every hour, assess lung sounds, observe for chest retractions, and check bilateral peripheral pulses.
- Suction as needed to maintain airway patency, using sterile technique, providing adequate oxygen, and recording secretion characteristics, such as color, consistency, and amount.

- Ensure that the child receives chest physiotherapy and respiratory therapy every 4 hours.
- Monitor for signs of infection, such as fever, elevated white blood cell count, purulent sputum, or secretions.
- Use correct hand-washing technique and teach parents how to wash hands thoroughly before and after contact with the child.

NURSING DIAGNOSIS

Fluid volume excess related to the effects of BPD

DESIRED PATIENT OUTCOME

The child will maintain age-appropriate fluid volume

Outcome measurement criteria

☐ Age-appropriate vital signs

☐ Age-appropriate central venous pressure (CVP)

☐ Urine output of at least 1 ml/kg/hour

☐ Age-appropriate urine specific gravity

☐ Clear lung sounds

☐ Age-appropriate electrolyte values

☐ Absence of visible edema

Key interventions

- Monitor vital signs and electrocardiogram patterns continuously.
- Every hour, monitor CVP, auscultate lung sounds, and record urine output and specific gravity.
- Monitor and carefully document fluid intake and urine output.
- Monitor electrolyte values as prescribed.

- Inspect for edema every 8 hours and document findings.
- Administer medications as prescribed.

NURSING DIAGNOSIS

High risk for altered health maintenance related to insufficient knowledge of home care

DESIRED PATIENT OUTCOME

The parents will successfully manage the child's care

Outcome measurement criteria

- ☐ Verbalization by the parents of an understanding of BPD
- ☐ Verbalization by the parents of an understanding of the child's care
- ☐ Parental use of community support groups

Key interventions

- Explain the physical effects of the child's disease.
- Teach the parents how to use respiratory devices, such as a ventilator; administer medications and assess for their adverse effects; monitor food and fluid intake and output; and monitor for signs of infection, including changes in temperature, secretions, and respiratory effort. Stress the need for close follow-up care.
- Urge the parents to use community support groups and agencies.

NURSING DIAGNOSIS

High risk for caregiver role strain related to the complexity and long-term nature of care

DESIRED PATIENT OUTCOME

The parents will maintain optimum physical and mental health

Outcome measurement criteria

- □ Verbalization by the parents of a positive attitude toward the child
- □ Signs of physical and mental health of the parents
- □ Willingness of the parents to use support services
- □ Willingness of the parents to obtain respite care
- □ Demonstration of support by other family members

Key interventions

- Encourage the parents to discuss their feelings about care.
- Develop a plan in which family members share in care.
- Encourage the parents to have regular physical check-ups.
- Refer the parents to appropriate community support agencies and facilitate their use.
- Discuss the importance of the parents having a respite from care, such as an evening out or an occasional overnight trip.
- Encourage family members to provide mutual support, demonstrate caring attitudes, and acknowledge one another's contributions.

NURSING DIAGNOSIS

Altered nutrition: less than body requirements, related to increased energy needs

DESIRED PATIENT OUTCOME

The child will obtain sufficient nutrition to meet energy needs

Outcome measurement criteria

- ☐ Normal bowel sounds
- ☐ Balanced food and fluid intake and output
- ☐ Age-appropriate laboratory values
- ☐ Age-appropriate weight

Key interventions

- Auscultate bowel sounds before feeding.
- Consult with a dietitian and develop a high-protein, high-calorie diet.
- Monitor food and fluid intake and output.
- Monitor mineral and other laboratory test results to evaluate nutritional intake.
- Weigh the child daily if hospitalized and weekly if at home, at the same time, using the same scale, and with the child wearing the same amount of clothing.

Croup

Any of several acute viral syndromes that involve the upper and lower respiratory tract and range from mild to very severe. Croup syndromes include laryngotracheobronchitis, spasmodic laryngitis, acute epiglottitis, and acute tracheitis.

NURSING DIAGNOSIS

Anxiety related to breathing difficulty

DESIRED PATIENT OUTCOME

The child will resume normal breathing

Outcome measurement criteria

- ☐ Age-appropriate pulse and respiratory rates
- ☐ Absence of signs of respiratory distress
- ☐ Age-appropriate arterial blood gas (ABG) levels
- ☐ Verbalization by the parents of strategies that decrease respiratory difficulties
- ☐ Calm appearance of the child

Key interventions

- Monitor pulse and respiratory rates and auscultate the lungs.
- Administer aerosolized racemic epinephrine as prescribed. Note the child's response, including the pulse rate and breathing pattern. Prepare for cardiac monitoring if ordered.
- Assess for signs of respiratory distress, such as stridor, chest retractions, nasal flaring, use of accessory muscles, cyanosis, and anxiety.

- If the child reports a very sore throat, is drooling, or is sitting up and leaning forward, refrain from examining the throat; notify the primary care practitioner immediately, and prepare for endotracheal intubation or tracheostomy. These findings may signify acute epiglottitis.
- Monitor ABG levels.
- Provide a humidified environment with 40% oxygen.
- Provide I.V. hydration if respiratory distress is severe and continuous; administer fluids orally if the child desires and can tolerate them.
- Teach the parents strategies to use at home for mild croup, such as using a cool, moist vaporizer; taking the child into a steam-filled room, such as a bathroom in which a hot shower has been running; remaining calm in front of the child; and holding and comforting the child. Advise the parents to take the child to the emergency department if breathing becomes more labored.

Cystic fibrosis

Inherited disease of the exocrine glands and eccrine sweat glands that causes chronic respiratory infection, pancreatic insufficiency, abnormally thick mucus secretions, and susceptibility to thermal stress.

NURSING DIAGNOSIS

Ineffective airway clearance related to thick secretions

DESIRED PATIENT OUTCOME

The child will maintain a patent airway

Outcome measurement criteria

- ☐ Age-appropriate vital signs
- ☐ Absence of signs of acute respiratory distress
- ☐ Compliance with respiratory therapy regimen
- ☐ Arterial blood gas (ABG) levels within normal limits
- ☐ Age-appropriate hydration
- ☐ Verbalization by the parents of the child's home care needs
- ☐ Demonstration by the parents of the child's respiratory treatments

Key interventions

- Monitor temperature and pulse and respiratory rates every 4 hours, reporting elevations in vital signs.
- Auscultate the chest every 4 hours, noting any change in breath sounds.

- Record signs of respiratory distress, such as accessory muscle use, chest retractions, nasal flaring, wheezing, or cyanosis.
- Document the amount and characteristics of secretions, dispose of secretions appropriately, and report signs of infection to the primary care practitioner.
- Ensure that the respiratory therapist administers aerosol medications and treatments. Note the child's response.
- Administer oral and I.V. medications as prescribed, noting any reactions.
- Obtain specimens for ABG levels. Monitor ABG levels and notify the primary care practitioner if they are abnormal.
- Encourage the child to eat favorite fluids and provide snacks, such as gelatin, frozen pops, and juices.
- Teach the parents the importance of respiratory treatments and arrange for the respiratory therapist to teach them how to give breathing, percussion, and chest drainage treatments.
- Explain the administration, adverse effects, and signs of toxicity of such medications as bronchodilators and antibiotics.
- Discuss the signs of respiratory difficulty that indicate the child should see the primary care practitioner, including fever, increased difficulty with breathing, and rapid pulse or respiratory rate.
- Discuss the importance of exercise, stressing that exercise should be aerobic but not overly strenuous.

NURSING DIAGNOSIS

High risk for altered nutrition: less than body requirements, related to the effects of cystic fibrosis

DESIRED PATIENT OUTCOME

The child will maintain adequate nutrient intake

Outcome measurement criteria

- ☐ Verbalization by the parents and child (if age-appropriate) of the nutrients needed daily
- ☐ Compliance with medication regimen
- ☐ Age-appropriate weight and pulse rate
- ☐ Normal energy level
- ☐ Hemoglobin and hematocrit levels within normal limits
- ☐ Absence of steatorrhea
- ☐ Age-appropriate growth and development

Key interventions

- Consult the dietitian about the child's dietary needs.
- Teach the parents to administer the prescribed pancreatic enzymes with each meal and snack, sprinkled on food or swallowed in a capsule.
- Encourage the family to keep a record of the child's dietary intake, and review the record during follow-up visits. If intake is less than prescribed, arrange for another consultation with the dietitian.
- Assess the child's food preferences, encouraging the child to eat nutritionally sound, favorite foods. Provide high-carbohydrate snacks.
- Monitor the child's weight during follow-up visits; encourage the parents to weigh the child weekly and to report weight loss.
- Ask the parents about the child's energy level, discussing signs of activity intolerance, such as increased pulse and respiratory rates, and ways to conserve the child's energy.
- Monitor hemoglobin and hematocrit levels.

- Monitor the amount of steatorrhea and the number of bowel movements daily. Be aware that the amount of pancreatic enzyme may have to be adjusted.
- Monitor the child's growth using age-appropriate norms. Assess social, language, and motor development.

NURSING DIAGNOSIS

High risk for caregiver role strain related to the complexity and long-term nature of care

DESIRED PATIENT OUTCOME

The parents will maintain optimum physical and mental health

Outcome measurement criteria

- ☐ Verbalization by the parents of a positive attitude toward the child and care responsibilities
- ☐ Signs of physical and mental health of the parents
- ☐ Willingness of the parents to use support services
- ☐ Willingness of the parents to obtain respite care
- ☐ Demonstration of support by other family members

Key interventions

- Encourage the parents to discuss feelings about care.
- Encourage the parents to have regular checkups.
- Refer the parents to appropriate community support agencies and facilitate their use. Discuss the importance of having a respite from care, such as an evening out.
- Develop a plan in which family members share care.
- Encourage family members to provide mutual support and demonstrate caring attitudes.

Respiratory infection, acute

Abrupt onset of signs and symptoms of invasion of the upper or lower respiratory tract by pathogens, such as Staphylococcus *and respiratory syncytial virus.*

NURSING DIAGNOSIS

Ineffective breathing pattern related to the effects of respiratory infection

DESIRED PATIENT OUTCOME

The child will display a normal breathing pattern

Outcome measurement criteria

- □ Age-appropriate pulse and respiratory rates
- □ Clear breath sounds
- □ Absence of nasal flaring
- □ Symmetrical chest expansion
- □ Absence of chest retractions
- □ Age-appropriate ABG levels
- □ Normal energy level

Key interventions

- Monitor pulse and respiratory rates and auscultate the lungs every 4 hours.
- Note nasal flaring. Inspect the chest for symmetrical expansion; observe for retractions.
- Clear nasal passages of secretions by suctioning with a bulb syringe.
- Monitor ABG levels and notify the primary care practitioner of abnormal levels.

- Provide humidified oxygen as prescribed, using an age-appropriate delivery method.
- Assure that respiratory treatments are administered at appropriate times.
- Note the child's energy level, and organize care so the child has undisturbed rest periods.

NURSING DIAGNOSIS

High risk for altered body temperature related to the effects of respiratory infection

DESIRED PATIENT OUTCOME

The child will display a normal body temperature

Outcome measurement criteria

- ☐ Oral or tympanic temperature of 99° F (37.2° C) or less; axillary temperature of 98° F (36.7° C) or less
- ☐ Normal breath sounds
- ☐ Lung free from signs of infection
- ☐ Absence of signs of pharyngeal infection
- ☐ Negative results on pharyngeal culture
- ☐ Age-appropriate white blood cell (WBC) count

Key interventions

- Monitor the child's temperature every 4 hours.
- Administer acetaminophen or other medication, as prescribed, for an oral or tympanic temperature at or above 101° F (38.3° C) or for an axillary temperature at or above 100° F (37.7° C) Avoid using aspirin if a viral disease is suspected.
- Keep minimal clothing on the child, being careful not to chill the child. Keep the room temperature cool but comfortable.

- Check the record for a history of febrile seizures; if present, take seizure precautions.
- Auscultate breath sounds, noting diminished or abnormal sounds.
- Ensure that chest X-rays are taken and that results are noted on the chart. Notify the primary care practitioner of results.
- Ask the child about pharyngeal discomfort. Do not examine or culture the pharynx if severe discomfort or drooling is present.
- Obtain a pharyngeal culture specimen if ordered, noting the results and conveying them to the primary care practitioner.
- Monitor the WBC count.

NURSING DIAGNOSIS

High risk for fluid volume deficit related to insufficient intake

DESIRED PATIENT OUTCOME

The child will maintain an age-appropriate fluid intake

Outcome measurement criteria

☐ Age-appropriate fluid intake

☐ Adequate urine output (1 to 2 ml/kg/hour)

☐ Age-appropriate urine specific gravity

☐ Elastic skin turgor

☐ Moist mucous membranes

☐ Age-appropriate vital signs

☐ Capillary refill time of less than 2 seconds

☐ Flat (not depressed) anterior fontanel, if patent

☐ Serum electrolyte and pH levels within normal ranges

- ☐ Verbalization by the parents of ways to maintain hydration at home

Key interventions

- Carefully document fluid intake and urine output.
- Monitor the I.V. site for edema, redness, or pain and monitor the I.V. solution and drip rate for accuracy, using an electronic I.V. monitor.
- Encourage consumption of favorite fluids, note fluid tolerance, and use gelatin and frozen pops as alternatives to drinks.
- Weigh diapers if the child normally wears them, or enlist the parents' help in measuring urine output if the child is toilet trained. Check urine specific gravity every 4 hours.
- Every 4 hours, check skin turgor, assess mucous membrane moistness, monitor vital signs, and check the capillary refill time of the nails.
- Check the anterior fontanel, if patent, and notify the primary care practitioner if it is depressed or bulging.
- Monitor serum electrolyte and pH levels, notifying the primary care practitioner of abnormal levels.
- Teach the parents how to keep the child hydrated when at home with a respiratory illness, including keeping the child's temperature within the normal range by using acetaminophen; keeping the room cool; avoiding excessive clothing or covers; offering small, frequent drinks of favorite fluids; tempting the child with frozen pops or gelatin; and checking to ensure that the child is urinating.

NURSING DIAGNOSIS

High risk for altered nutrition: less than body requirements, related to anorexia

DESIRED PATIENT OUTCOME

The child will maintain age-appropriate nutritional intake

Outcome measurement criteria

- Age-appropriate weight
- Laboratory test results indicating adequate nutrient intake
- Verbalization by the parents of the importance of adequate nutritional intake

Key interventions

- Weigh the child daily at the same time, using the same scale, and with the child wearing the same amount of clothing. Compare the present weight with the child's preillness weight.
- Provide high-calorie food and fluids, gradually returning the child to an age-appropriate diet.
- Monitor laboratory test results, alerting the primary care practitioner of abnormalities.
- Teach the parents the age-appropriate diet for the child, discussing the relationship between adequate nutrient intake, health, and the child's ability to recover from illness.

APPENDIX 1

NANDA taxonomy of nursing diagnoses

The currently accepted classification system for nursing diagnoses is that of the North American Nursing Diagnosis Association (NANDA), as shown in *NANDA Nursing Diagnoses: Definitions and Classification 1992-1993*. It is organized around nine human response patterns: exchanging, communicating, relating, valuing, choosing, moving, perceiving, knowing, and feeling.

The complete taxonomic structure is listed here. The series of numbers before each diagnosis is its classification number, used to determine the placement of the diagnosis within the taxonomy. The number of digits delineates the level of abstraction of the nursing diagnosis (more specific diagnoses are assigned longer numbers).

Pattern 1. Exchanging

1.1.2.1	Altered nutrition: More than body requirements
1.1.2.2	Altered nutrition: Less than body requirements
1.1.2.3	Altered nutrition: Potential for more than body requirements
1.2.1.1	High risk for infection
1.2.2.1	High risk for altered body temperature
1.2.2.2	Hypothermia
1.2.2.3	Hyperthermia
1.2.2.4	Ineffective thermoregulation
1.2.3.1	Dysreflexia
1.3.1.1	Constipation
1.3.1.1.1	Perceived constipation
1.3.1.1.2	Colonic constipation
1.3.1.2	Diarrhea
1.3.1.3	Bowel incontinence
1.3.2	Altered urinary elimination
1.3.2.1.1	Stress incontinence
1.3.2.1.2	Reflex incontinence
1.3.2.1.3	Urge incontinence
1.3.2.1.4	Functional incontinence
1.3.2.1.5	Total incontinence
1.3.2.2	Urinary retention
1.4.1.1	Altered (specify type) tissue perfusion (renal, cerebral, cardiopulmonary, gastrointestinal, peripheral)
1.4.1.2.1	Fluid volume excess
1.4.1.2.2.1	Fluid volume deficit
1.4.1.2.2.2	High risk for fluid volume deficit
1.4.2.1	Decreased cardiac output
1.5.1.1	Impaired gas exchange
1.5.1.2	Ineffective airway clearance
1.5.1.3	Ineffective breathing pattern
1.5.1.3.1	Inability to sustain spontaneous ventilation
1.5.1.3.2	Dysfunctional ventilatory weaning response
1.6.1	High risk for injury
1.6.1.1	High risk for suffocation
1.6.1.2	High risk for poisoning
1.6.1.3	High risk for trauma
1.6.1.4	High risk for aspiration
1.6.1.5	High risk for disuse syndrome
1.6.2	Altered protection
1.6.2.1	Impaired tissue integrity
1.6.2.1.1	Altered oral mucous membrane
1.6.2.1.2.1	Impaired skin integrity
1.6.2.1.2.2	High risk for impaired skin integrity

Pattern 2. Communicating

2.1.1.1	Impaired verbal communication

Pattern 3. Relating

3.1.1	Impaired social interaction
3.1.2	Social isolation
3.2.1	Altered role performance
3.2.1.1.1	Altered parenting
3.2.1.1.2	High risk for altered parenting
3.2.1.2.1	Sexual dysfunction
3.2.2	Altered family processes
3.2.2.1	Caregiver role strain
3.2.2.2	High risk for caregiver role strain
3.2.3.1	Parental role conflict
3.3	Altered sexuality patterns

Pattern 4. Valuing

4.1.1 Spiritual distress (distress of the human spirit)

Pattern 5. Choosing

5.1.1.1 Ineffective individual coping
5.1.1.1.1 Impaired adjustment
5.1.1.1.2 Defensive coping
5.1.1.1.3 Ineffective denial
5.1.2.1.1 Ineffective family coping: Disabling
5.1.2.1.2 Ineffective family coping: Compromised
5.1.2.2 Family coping: Potential for growth
5.2.1 Ineffective management of therapeutic regimen (individual)
5.2.1.1 Noncompliance (specify)
5.3.1.1 Decisional conflict (specify)
5.4 Health-seeking behaviors (specify)

Pattern 6. Moving

6.1.1.1 Impaired physical mobility
6.1.1.1.1 High risk for peripheral neurovascular dysfunction
6.1.1.2 Activity intolerance
6.1.1.2.1 Fatigue
6.1.1.3 High risk for activity intolerance
6.2.1 Sleep pattern disturbance
6.3.1.1 Diversional activity deficit
6.4.1.1 Impaired home maintenance management
6.4.2 Altered health maintenance
6.5.1 Feeding self-care deficit
6.5.1.1 Impaired swallowing
6.5.1.2 Ineffective breast-feeding
6.5.1.2.1 Interrupted breast-feeding
6.5.1.3 Effective breast-feeding
6.5.1.4 Ineffective infant feeding pattern
6.5.2 Bathing or hygiene self-care deficit
6.5.3 Dressing or grooming self-care deficit
6.5.4 Toileting self-care deficit
6.6 Altered growth and development
6.7 Relocation stress syndrome

Pattern 7. Perceiving

7.1.1 Body image disturbance
7.1.2 Self-esteem disturbance
7.1.2.1 Chronic low self-esteem
7.1.2.2 Situational low self-esteem
7.1.3 Personal identity disturbance
7.2 Sensory or perceptual alterations (specify visual, auditory, kinesthetic, gustatory, tactile, olfactory)
7.2.1.1 Unilateral neglect
7.3.1 Hopelessness
7.3.2 Powerlessness

Pattern 8. Knowing

8.1.1 Knowledge deficit (specify)
8.3 Altered thought processes

Pattern 9. Feeling

9.1.1 Pain
9.1.1.1 Chronic pain
9.2.1.1 Dysfunctional grieving
9.2.1.2 Anticipatory grieving
9.2.2 High risk for violence: Self-directed or directed at others
9.2.2.1 High risk for self-mutilation
9.2.3 Post-trauma response
9.2.3.1 Rape-trauma syndrome
9.2.3.1.1 Rape-trauma syndrome: Compound reaction
9.2.3.1.2 Rape-trauma syndrome: Silent reaction
9.3.1 Anxiety
9.3.2 Fear

APPENDIX 2

Common nursing diagnoses in pediatric care

The following list summarizes the nursing diagnoses that appear in this book, which are among the most common diagnoses in pediatric care.

ACCIDENTS, INCIDENTS, AND INFECTIONS

Burns

- Ineffective airway clearance related to upper airway inflammation and edema
- Fluid volume deficit related to burn-induced fluid loss and interstitial fluid shift
- Altered nutrition: less than body requirements, related to poor intake and increased metabolic needs
- Impaired physical mobility related to acute pain secondary to the injury and therapy
- High risk for infection related to loss of skin secondary to a burn
- Altered family processes related to the child's hospitalization and probable long-term rehabilitation
- High risk for injury related to lack of knowledge about preventing burns

Childhood communicable diseases

- High risk for fluid volume deficit related to fever or decreased oral intake
- High risk for infection (in others) related to lack of knowledge about transmission prevention
- Altered comfort related to pruritus
- Altered health maintenance related to lack of knowledge about immunization schedule

Foreign body aspiration

- Ineffective airway clearance related to obstruction by a foreign body
- High risk for aspiration related to lack of knowledge about preventing foreign body aspiration

Infectious lesions

- High risk for infection (in others) related to lack of knowledge about the condition and its prevention

Infectious mononucleosis

- Altered health maintenance related to lack of knowledge about mononucleosis

Insect infestation

- High risk for infection (in others) related to lack of knowledge about the condition and transmission prevention
- High risk for infection (secondary) related to pruritus

Poisoning, acute

- High risk for poisoning related to insufficient parental knowledge about poisoning prevention
- High risk for injury related to insufficient parental knowledge about first aid for accidental poisoning
- Anxiety (parental) related to uncertainty about the outcome of the child's poisoning

Stings and bites

- Impaired tissue integrity related to stings and bites

Sudden infant death syndrome

- Altered family processes related to an infant's death caused by sudden infant death syndrome (SIDS)

CARDIOVASCULAR DISORDERS

Cardiac catheterization

- Anxiety related to lack of knowledge about the cardiac catheterization procedure and home care
- High risk for infection related to wound and cardiac catheterization

Congestive heart failure

- Activity intolerance related to insufficient oxygen supply secondary to congestive heart failure (CHF)
- High risk for ineffective management of therapeutic regimen (parental) related to the complexity of the regimen to treat CHF

Heart defects, congenital

- Anxiety related to lack of knowledge about surgery for congenital heart defects
- Anxiety related to the unknown outcome of surgery for congenital heart defects
- Ineffective breathing pattern related to the effects of surgery for congenital heart defects
- Fluid volume deficit related to surgery for congenital heart defects
- Pain related to tissue trauma secondary to chest surgery and hospitalization
- Ineffective management of therapeutic regimen (parental) related to the complexity of the regimen after surgical repair of congenital heart defects
- Altered family processes related to the requirements of caring for a child with congenital heart defects

Rheumatic fever, acute

- Anxiety related to lack of knowledge about acute rheumatic fever (ARF) and its treatment
- High risk for caregiver role strain related to lack of knowledge about ARF and the stress of caring for the child

CHRONIC DISORDERS

Chronic illness or impairment

- Anticipatory grieving related to loss of the child's health
- Anxiety related to lack of knowledge about the child's newly diagnosed illness or condition
- High risk for caregiver role strain related to the requirements of caring for a chronically ill or impaired child
- Feeding, bathing, hygiene, dressing, grooming, and toileting self-care deficits related to developmental delays secondary to chronic illness or impairment
- Altered growth and development related to frequent hospitalizations or treatments
- Pain related to treatments or procedures for or progression of a chronic illness or impairment
- Chronic low self-esteem related to lack of confidence caused by chronic illness or impairment

DEVELOPMENTAL CARE

Infant

- High risk for altered growth and development of the infant

Toddler or preschooler

- High risk for altered growth and development of the toddler or preschooler

School-age child

- High risk for altered growth and development of the school-age child

Adolescent

- High risk for altered growth and development of the adolescent

ENDOCRINE AND METABOLIC DISORDERS

Diabetes mellitus, insulin-dependent

- Anxiety related to lack of knowledge about diabetes mellitus
- Altered nutrition: less than body requirements, related to lack of knowledge about diet for diabetes mellitus
- High risk for injury related to insufficient glucose (hypoglycemia) or excessive glucose (hyperglycemia)
- High risk for caregiver role strain related to the stress of caring for a child with diabetes mellitus
- Altered growth and development related to the effects of hospitalization and treatment of diabetes mellitus

Hypothyroidism, congenital

- Anxiety related to insufficient parental knowledge about congenital hypothyroidism (CH)
- Altered health maintenance related to lack of parental knowledge about care of the child with CH

Phenylketonuria

- Anticipatory grieving (parental) related to the potential loss of the child's health because of phenylketonuria (PKU)
- Altered growth and development related to insufficient parental knowledge about PKU
- Altered health maintenance related to lack of knowledge about care of the child with PKU

EYE, EAR, NOSE, AND THROAT DISORDERS

Cleft lip and palate

- Anticipatory grieving (parental) related to loss of the child's health
- Altered parenting related to impaired parent-infant attachment
- Altered nutrition: less than body requirements, related to impaired feeding ability
- High risk for injury related to infection
- High risk for injury (to operative repair sites) related to the child's mobility and the parents' lack of knowledge about postoperative care
- High risk for caregiver role strain related to long-term home care

Communication or sensory impairment

- Impaired verbal communication related to articulation problems, sensory problems, or both

Myringotomy

- Anxiety related to lack of knowledge about myringotomy and follow-up care

Otitis media

- High risk for injury related to lack of parental knowledge about otitis media
- Pain related to pressure secondary to ear inflammation or infection

Tonsillectomy or adenoidectomy

- Anxiety related to lack of knowledge about the surgical procedure and postoperative care

GASTROINTESTINAL AND HEPATOBILIARY DISORDERS

Appendicitis, acute

- Anxiety related to lack of knowledge about preoperative procedures for appendectomy
- Pain related to inflammation secondary to incision for appendectomy
- High risk for infection related to disruption of skin integrity by the incision
- Fluid volume deficit related to nausea, vomiting, or both

Biliary atresia

- Anxiety (parental) related to lack of knowledge about biliary atresia and associated care
- Fluid volume deficit related to decreased absorption or excessive loss of nutrients

Esophageal atresia and tracheoesophageal fistula

- High risk for aspiration related to buildup of secretions
- Anxiety (parental) related to the consequences of the child's surgery
- Ineffective breathing pattern related to the effects of surgery for esophageal atresia and tracheoesophageal fistula
- Fluid volume deficit related to losses secondary to surgery for esophageal atresia and tracheoesophageal fistula
- Altered nutrition: less than body requirements, related to an alternative feeding method secondary to gastrostomy
- Pain related to tissue trauma secondary to surgery and hospitalization
- High risk for aspiration related to lack of knowledge about possible occlusion of the esophagus after surgical repair

Hepatitis

- Altered nutrition: less than body requirements, related to anorexia, loss of GI secretions, or malabsorption
- High risk for infection (in others) related to lack of knowledge about hepatitis
- Activity intolerance related to decreased energy
- High risk for injury related to medication ingestion during the acute stage of hepatitis

Hernia, inguinal or femoral

- Anxiety (parental) related to lack of knowledge about inguinal or femoral hernia and postoperative care

Liver transplant

- Ineffective family coping: compromised, related to uncertainty about a liver becoming available and the success of liver transplantation

Pyloric stenosis

- Anxiety (parental) related to lack of knowledge about pyloric stenosis and pyloroplasty
- Fluid volume deficit related to vomiting
- Altered nutrition: less than body requirements, related to the effects of surgery for pyloric stenosis
- Pain related to inflammation secondary to surgical incision to correct pyloric stenosis

Vomiting or diarrhea

- Fluid volume deficit related to increased loss of GI contents

GENERAL HOSPITAL CARE

General concerns related to hospitalization

- Anxiety related to the stresses of hospitalization
- Anxiety related to lack of knowledge about procedures
- High risk for ineffective family coping related to the effects of the child's hospitalization
- High risk for pain related to hospitalization experiences
- High risk for ineffective individual coping (child) related to the effects of hospitalization
- High risk for injury related to an unfamiliar environment
- Sensory or perceptual alterations (visual, auditory) related to the hospitalization experience
- Anxiety (parental) related to lack of knowledge of the child's condition or care

GENITOURINARY DISORDERS

Cryptorchidism

- Anxiety (parental) related to lack of knowledge about the child's condition
- Pain related to the effects of surgery to correct cryptorchidism
- High risk for fluid volume deficit related to the effects of surgery to correct cryptorchidism
- High risk for infection related to the effects of the surgical incision's location

Glomerulonephritis, acute

- Anxiety (parental) related to lack of knowledge about acute glomerulonephritis
- Fluid volume excess related to the effects of acute glomerulonephritis
- Altered nutrition: less than body requirements, related to anorexia

Hydrocele

- Anxiety (parental) related to lack of knowledge about hydrocele and related infant care

Hypospadias or epispadias

- High risk for dysfunctional grieving (parental) related to loss of the infant's health
- Anxiety (parental) related to lack of knowledge about surgery for hypospadias or epispadias and related care
- High risk for injury (to the surgical site) related to activity after surgery

Kidney transplant

- Anxiety (parental, child) related to lack of knowledge about and preparation for kidney transplantation
- High risk for altered health maintenance related to insufficient knowledge about managing the treatment regimen

Nephrotic syndrome

- Fluid volume excess related to the effects of nephrotic syndrome
- Altered nutrition: less than body requirements, related to anorexia
- Fatigue related to the effects of nephrotic syndrome
- High risk for infection related to the effects of nephrotic syndrome and its treatment
- High risk for ineffective management of therapeutic regimen (parental) related to lack of knowledge about nephrotic syndrome and related home care

Ureteral reimplantation

- Anxiety (parental, child) related to lack of knowledge about the child's condition and treatment
- Pain related to the effects of the surgical incision and related procedures
- High risk for infection related to the surgical incision and urinary diversion devices

HEMATOLOGIC AND IMMUNOLOGIC DISORDERS

Acquired immunodeficiency syndrome

- Fear (parental, child) related to the effects of acquired immunodeficiency syndrome (AIDS) and its fatal prognosis
- High risk for infection related to a compromised immune system
- High risk for altered health maintenance related to the complexity of the care regimen

Hemophilia A

- Anxiety (parental) related to lack of knowledge about the child's condition
- High risk for altered health maintenance related to the effects of the child's newly diagnosed hemophilia A
- Pain related to the effects of bleeding into tissues

Iron deficiency anemia

- Altered health maintenance related to lack of knowledge about appropriate dietary iron intake

Leukemia

- Anxiety (parental) related to lack of knowledge about the child's condition and prognosis
- Altered protection related to the body's decreased defenses
- Altered protection related to the response to chemotherapy
- Altered nutrition: less than body requirements, related to the effects of chemotherapy

Shock

- Fluid volume deficit related to blood loss
- High risk for altered body temperature related to the effects of systemic infection
- Ineffective breathing pattern related to the effects of shock
- High risk for injury (complications) related to ischemia

Sickle cell anemia

- Anxiety (parental) related to lack of knowledge about the child's condition and care
- Pain related to the effects of cell sickling
- High risk for fluid volume deficit related to the effects of infection

MUSCULOSKELETAL DISORDERS

Clubfoot, congenital

- High risk for impaired skin integrity related to the effects of wearing a cast or Denis Browne splint
- High risk for altered growth and development related to immobilization

Fracture

- Pain related to the effects of bone trauma or disease
- High risk for impaired skin integrity related to lack of parental knowledge about required care

Hip dysplasia, congenital

- Altered peripheral tissue perfusion related to immobility
- High risk for impaired skin integrity related to the parents' lack of knowledge about the child's disorder
- High risk for altered growth and development related to the effects of wearing a cast or other corrective device

Osteomyelitis

- Pain related to the effects of osteomyelitis
- High risk for altered growth and development related to the effects of long-term antibiotic treatment for osteomyelitis

Rheumatoid arthritis, juvenile

- Pain related to inflammation associated with juvenile rheumatoid arthritis
- High risk for activity intolerance related to pain and fatigue secondary to juvenile rheumatoid arthritis
- High risk for altered health maintenance related to insufficient knowledge about home care

Scoliosis

- Anxiety related to lack of knowledge about scoliosis and its outcome
- Pain related to the effects of surgery for scoliosis
- High risk for altered health maintenance related to concerns secondary to adolescence

NEUROLOGIC DISORDERS

Cerebral palsy

- Grieving (parental) related to loss of the child's health
- Anxiety (parental) related to lack of knowledge about cerebral palsy and required care
- High risk for altered nutrition: less than body requirements, related to difficulty with sucking and swallowing
- High risk for impaired home maintenance management related to the complexity of care
- High risk for body image disturbance related to the effects of cerebral palsy

Head trauma

- High risk for injury related to the effects of head trauma
- High risk for altered health maintenance related to lack of knowledge about caring for the child with head trauma

Hydrocephalus

- High risk for injury related to the effects of hydrocephalus
- Anxiety (parental) related to lack of knowledge about hydrocephalus and related home care
- High risk for caregiver role strain related to the demands of long-term care

Myelomeningocele

- Anxiety (parental) related to lack of knowledge about the disorder
- Grieving (parental) related to loss of the child's health
- High risk for infection related to the effects of a spinal defect
- Impaired physical mobility related to the effects of myelomeningocele
- High risk for caregiver role strain related to the complexity of long-term care

Reye's syndrome

- Anxiety (parental) related to the uncertainty of the disorder's outcome
- High risk for injury related to the effects of Reye's syndrome

Seizures

- Altered protection related to seizures
- High risk for social isolation related to fear of having a seizure

PSYCHOSOCIAL AND MENTAL DISORDERS

Anorexia nervosa or bulimia nervosa

- Altered nutrition: less than body requirements, related to aversion to weight gain or self-induced vomiting and laxative abuse
- Body image disturbance related to perception of self as obese

Autism, infantile

- Impaired social interaction related to the effects of autism
- High risk for self-mutilation related to the effects of autism

Child abuse or neglect

- Fear (child) related to removal from the parents
- Ineffective individual coping (nonabusing parent) related to fear of the abuser
- Ineffective family coping: disabling, related to situational factors
- High risk for altered health maintenance related to insufficient parenting skills

Depression

- Ineffective individual coping related to low self-esteem and situational stressors
- High risk for social isolation related to feelings of hopelessness and worthlessness
- High risk for altered nutrition: less than body requirements, related to inappropriate eating patterns
- Sleep pattern disturbance related to emotional stress
- High risk for violence: self-directed, related to situational factors

Failure to thrive, inorganic

- Altered parenting related to lack of knowledge about parenting skills
- Altered nutrition: less than body requirements, related to inadequate food intake

Mental retardation

- Grieving (parental) related to loss of the child's mental health
- Anxiety related to lack of knowledge about mental retardation
- High risk for feeding, bathing, hygiene, dressing, and grooming self-care deficits related to impaired cognitive functioning
- High risk for caregiver role strain related to the demands of caring for a mentally retarded child

Obesity

- Ineffective individual coping related to increased food consumption
- Altered health maintenance related to lack of knowledge about exercise and diet
- High risk for social isolation related to fear of negative responses from others

Schizophrenia

- Impaired verbal communication related to the effects of schizophrenia and its treatment
- Impaired social interaction related to the effects of schizophrenia

RESPIRATORY DISORDERS

Asthma

- High risk for ineffective breathing pattern related to lack of knowledge about asthma and its management
- Ineffective breathing pattern related to increased mucus production and narrowed respiratory passages
- High risk for caregiver role strain related to the stress of caring for a chronically ill child

Bronchopulmonary dysplasia

- Impaired gas exchange related to the effects of bronchopulmonary dysplasia (BPD)
- Fluid volume excess related to the effects of BPD
- High risk for altered health maintenance related to insufficient knowledge of home care
- High risk for caregiver role strain related to the complexity and long-term nature of care
- Altered nutrition: less than body requirements, related to increased energy needs

Croup

- Anxiety related to breathing difficulty

Cystic fibrosis

- Ineffective airway clearance related to thick secretions
- High risk for altered nutrition: less than body requirements, related to the effects of cystic fibrosis
- High risk for caregiver role strain related to the complexity and long-term nature of care

Respiratory infection, acute

- Ineffective breathing pattern related to the effects of respiratory infection
- High risk for altered body temperature related to the effects of respiratory infection
- High risk for fluid volume deficit related to insufficient intake
- High risk for altered nutrition: less than body requirements, related to anorexia

SELECTED REFERENCES

Books

Axton, S., and Fugate, T. (1993). Pediatric care plans. Redwood City, CA: Addison-Wesley Publishing Co.

Gulanick, M., Puzas, M., and Wilson, C. (1992). Nursing care plans for newborns and children: Acute and critical care. St. Louis: Mosby-Year Book.

Iyer, P., Taptich, B., and Losey, D. (1994). Nursing process and nursing diagnosis (3rd ed.). Philadelphia: W.B. Saunders Co.

McFarland, G., and Wasli, E. (1992). Nursing diagnosis and process: Psychiatric mental health (2nd ed.). Philadelphia: J.B. Lippincott Co.

Phipps, W. (1991). Medical surgical nursing: Concepts and clinical practice (4th ed.). St. Louis: Mosby-Year Book.

Skale, N. (1992). Manual of pediatric nursing procedures. Philadelphia: J.B. Lippincott Co.

Sparks, S., and Taylor, C. (1993). Nursing diagnosis reference manual (2nd ed.). Springhouse, PA: Springhouse Corp.

Speer, K., and Swann, C. (1993). The Addison-Wesley manual of pediatric nursing procedures. Redwood City, CA: Addison-Wesley Publishing Co.

Townsend, M. (1993). Psychiatric-mental health nursing: Concepts of care. Philadelphia: F.A. Davis Co.

Williams, B., and Baer, C. (1994). Essentials of clinical pharmacology and nursing (2nd ed.). Springhouse, PA: Springhouse Corp.

Wong, D., and Whaley, L. (1992). Whaley and Wong's Essentials of Pediatric nursing (4th ed.). St. Louis: Mosby-Year Book.

Periodicals

Andrus, C. (1991). Intracranial pressure: Dynamics and nursing management. *Journal of Neuroscience Nursing,* 23(2), 85-92.

Brandt, P., and Magyary, D. (1993). The impact of a diabetes education program on children and mothers. *Journal of Pediatric Nursing,* 8(1), 31-40.

Breitmayer, B., Gallo, A., Knafl, K., and Zoeller, L. (1992). Social competence of school-aged children with chronic illnesses. *Journal of Pediatric Nursing,* 7(3), 181-188.

Carabott, J., Javaheri, Z., Keilty, K., and Manger, G. (1992). Oral fluid intake in children following tonsillectomy and adenoidectomy. *Pediatric Nursing,* 18(2), 124-127.

Davis, B., and Steele, S. (1991). Case management for young children with special health care needs. *Pediatric Nursing,* 17(1), 15-27.

Devlin, B., and Reynolds, E. (1994) Child abuse: How to recognize it, how to intervene. *American Journal of Nursing,* 94(3), 26-31.

DiMola, M. (1993). The cutting edge in burn care. *Critical Care Nurse,* Suppl., 24-30.

Faux, S. (1991). Sibling relationships in families with congenitally impaired children. *Journal of Pediatric Nursing,* 6(3), 175-184.

Fosdal, M. (1992). Living with spina bifida. *Journal of Neuroscience Nursing,* 24(5), 286-289.

George, A., and Hancock, J. (1993). Reducing pediatric burn pain with parent participation. *Journal of Burn Care and Rehabilitation,* 14(1), 104-107.

Herman-Staab, B. (1992). Antecedents to nonorganic failure-to-thrive. *Pediatric Nursing,* 18(6), 579-590.

HIV Guideline Panel. (1994). Quick reference guide for clinicians managing early HIV infection. *Journal of the American Academy of Nursing Practitioners,* 6(2), 65-82.

Kirk, E., White, C., and Freeman, S. (1992). Effects of a nursing education intervention on parents' knowledge of hydrocephalus and shunts. *Journal of Neuroscience Nursing,* 24(2), 99-103.

Klein, E. (1992). Premedicating children for painful invasive procedures. *Journal of Pediatric Oncology Nursing,* 9(4), 170-179.

Kyzer, S. (1991). Congenital idiopathic clubfoot. *Orthopaedic Nursing,* 10(4), 11-32.

Lindgren, C., Burke, M., Hainsworth, M., and Eakes, G. (1992). Chronic sorrow: A lifespan concept. *Scholarly Inquiry for Nursing Practice,* 6(1), 27-42.

Loutzenhiser, J., and Clark, R. (1993). Physical activity and exercise in children with cystic fibrosis. *Journal of Pediatric Nursing,* 8(2), 112-119.

Martinez, N., Schreiber, M., and Hartman, E. (1991.) Pediatric nurse practitioners: Primary care providers and case managers for chronically ill children at home. *Journal of Pediatric Health Care,* 5(6), 291-298.

Mayhew, M. (1991). Strategies for promoting safety and preventing injury. *Nursing Clinics of North America,* 26(4), 885-893.

McIntosh, K. (1993). Respiratory syncytial virus: Successful immunoprophylaxis at last. *The New England Journal of Medicine,* 329(21), 1572-1573.

Meyer-Pahoulis, E., et al. (1993). The pediatric patient in the post anesthesia care unit. *Nursing Clinics of North America,* 28(3), 519-530.

Morelli, J. (1993). Pediatric poisonings: The 10 most toxic prescription drugs. *American Journal of Nursing,* 93(7), 26-29.

Moscicki, A., Millstein, S., Broering, J., and Irwin, C. (1993). Risks of human immunodeficiency virus infection among adolescents attending three diverse clinics. *Journal of Pediatrics,* 122(5, part 1), 813-820.

Pasero, C., and McCaffery, M. (1993). Unconventional PCA: Making it work for your patient. *American Journal of Nursing,* 93(9), 38-41.

Reishtein, J. (1993). Liver failure: Case study of a complex problem. *Critical Care Nursing,* 13(5), 36-47.

Richard, M. (1991). Feeding the newborn with cleft lip and/or palate: The enlargement, stimulate, swallow, rest (ESSR) method. *Journal of Pediatric Nursing,* 6(5), 317-321.

Rose, B. (1993). Neurologic therapies in critical care. *Critical Care Nursing Clinics of North America,* 5(2), 237-246.

Schmidt, K., et al. (1994). How to apply the AHCPR's pediatric pain guideline. *American Journal of Nursing,* 94(3), 69-74.

Semonin-Holleran, R. (1993). Taking the sting out of summer. *RN,* 56(7), 40-46.

Shantz, D., and Spitz, M. (1993). What you need to know about seizures. *Nursing93,* 23(11), 34-46.

Sherman, J., et al. (1992). Intervention program for obese school children. *Journal of Community Health Nursing,* 9(3), 183-190.

Smith, K. (1991). Bowel and bladder management of the child with myelomeningocele in the school setting. *Journal of Enterostomal Therapy,* 18(1), 6-10.

Wagner, J., and Menke, E. (1991). The depression of homeless children: A focus for nursing intervention. *Issues in Comprehensive Pediatric Nursing,* 14(1), 17-29.

INDEX

A

B

C

D

E

F

G

H

I